The Complete

Gout-Friendly

Cookbook for Seniors

Easy Low-Purine Recipes to Reduce Uric Acid, Inflammation, Manage Flares & Live a Vibrant Life

Grace N. Rodney

Copyright © 2024 by Grace N. Rodney

All rights reserved. No part of this publication may be reproduced, distributed, or transmitted in any form or by any means, including photocopying, recording, or other electronic or mechanical methods, without the prior written permission of the publisher, except in the case of brief quotations embodied in critical reviews and certain other noncommercial uses permitted by copyright law.

Disclaimer:

The information provided in this book is intended for general knowledge and informational purposes only, and does not constitute medical advice. It is essential to consult with a qualified healthcare professional for any health concerns or before making any decisions related to your health or treatment. The author and publisher disclaim any liability for any adverse effects or consequences resulting from the use of the information or recipes provided in this book.

TABLE OF CONTENTS

Introduction 6

Chapter 1: Understanding Gout in Older Adults 8

    1.1   What is Gout 8

    1.2   How Gout Attacks Develop 9

    1.3. Risk Factors for Gout 10

Chapter 2: Diagnosis and Treatment of Gout 12

    2.1   Diagnostic tests for gout 12

    2.2   Conventional treatment options for gout 13

    2.3   Medications to Prevent Gout Complications 15

Chapter 3: The Gout Diet Explained 16

    3.1   The role of purines in gout 16

    3.3   Benefits of following a gout diet 17

    3.2   Foods high, moderate, and low in purines 18

    3.4   Nutritional considerations for seniors with gout 19

    3.5   Medication interactions with food 20

Delicious and Easy Gout-Friendly Recipes for Seniors 22

Chapter 4: Breakfast Recipes 22

    Greek Yogurt with Fresh Fruit, Chia Seeds, & Almonds 23

    Avocado Toast with Tomato, Basil, and Smoked Salmon 24

    Grapefruit and Cottage Cheese with Mixed Nuts 25

    Whole Wheat Toast with Natural Peanut Butter, Banana, and Chia Seeds 26

Spinach and Feta Stuffed Mushrooms with Quinoa 27

Baked Oatmeal with Blueberries, Almonds, and Greek Yogurt 28

Veggie Omelet with Goat Cheese and Fresh Herbs 29

Overnight Oats with Berries, Walnuts, and Protein Powder............................. 30

Quinoa Porridge with Cinnamon, Apples, and Flaxseed...................................... 31

Egg White Veggie Frittata with Kale and Fresh Herbs.. 32

Chapter 5: Lunch Recipes (Light and satisfying meals).. 34

Whole Grain Chicken Spinach Mushroom Flatbread 35

Beef & Barley Soup with Leafy Greens 36

Salad with Cheese, Avocado, and Hard-Boiled Egg 37

Whole Grain Ham and Cheese Panini 38

Turkey, Avocado, and Tomato Wrap with Spinach.. 39

Vegetable Omelet with Feta Cheese 40

Whole Wheat Mac 'n Cheese with Ham and Broccoli 41

Roast Chicken with Garlic Potatoes and Glazed Carrots................................ 42

Baked Salmon with Quinoa and Steamed Broccoli 43

Hearty Beef and Root Vegetable Stew... 44

Chapter 6: Dinner Recipes (Hearty and flavorful dishes).. 46

Marinated Baked Salmon with Herb-Roasted Vegetables 46

Lean Chicken and Broccoli Stir-Fry 47

Flavorful Lentil and Sweet Potato Curry 49

Lean Beef and Barley Soup.. 50

Stuffed Bell Peppers with Turkey and Quinoa 52

Tuna Salad Lettuce Wraps with Crunchy Vegetables 54

Baked Cod with Almond-Herb Topping 55

Vegetable Frittata with Feta and Spinach 56

Turkey Meatballs with Whole Wheat Pasta and Steamed Broccoli 57

Creamy Butternut Squash Soup with Toasted Pumpkin Seeds 58

Chapter 7: Side Dish and Snack Recipes (Healthy and enjoyable options) 60

Spiced Roasted Chickpeas 61

Caprese Skewers with Balsamic Drizzle 62

Greek Yogurt Dip with Crunchy Veggies 62

Quinoa and Feta Stuffed Bell Peppers 63

Fruit Salad with Honey-Lime Dressing 64

Cucumber Avocado Rolls with Herbs 65

Crispy Baked Sweet Potato Fries 66

Edamame with Lemon Pepper Seasoning 67

Mango Salsa with Whole Grain Pita Chips 68

Spinach and Feta Stuffed Mushrooms 69

Chapter 8: Dessert Recipes (Sweet treats without compromising gout management) 70

Easy Applesauce 71

Graham Cracker Delight 72

Lazy Apple Crisp 73

Berry Cherry Smoothie 74

Gooey Blueberry Oat Bars 75

Chocolate Covered Strawberries 76

Better-for-You Peanut Butter Brownies 77

Creamy Avocado Pudding 78

Pistachio Cranberry Dark Chocolate Bark 79

Cast Iron Mango and Peach Cobbler 80

Chapter 9: Maintaining a Healthy Weight for Gout Control 82

The Prevalence of Gout in Older Adults 82

Safe and effective weight loss strategies for seniors 85

Chapter 10: Exercise and Physicala Activity 88

Why Exercise Matters 88

Gout-Friendly Exercise Options 88

Staying Active with Joint Limitations 89

Chapter 11: Hydration and Lifestyle Habits for Healthy Aging with Gout 90

Importance of Staying Hydrated for Gout Sufferers 90

Stress Management Techniques for Seniors with Gout 91

Importance of Good Sleep for Overall Health 91

28-Day Meal Plan 94

Gout-Friendly Weekly Shopping List 97

Bonus Section 100

Conclusion 106

Introduction

Have you ever woken up in the agony of a gout flare-up? Simple tasks like getting dressed or reaching for that morning cup of coffee suddenly become major challenges. The throbbing pain in your toe makes even standing unbearable, and the thought of chopping vegetables feels like an impossible feat.

Did you know that gout affects nearly 1 in 25 seniors in the United States? It can rob you of your independence and make even the most basic activities feel overwhelming.

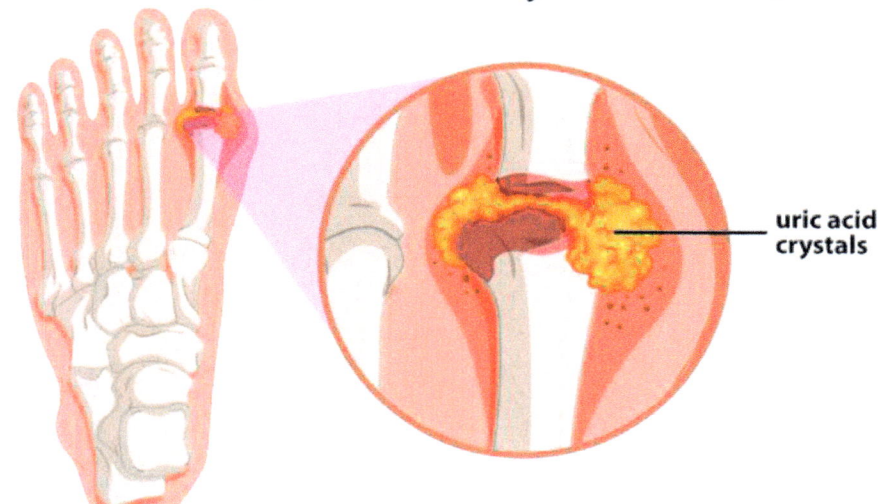

But here's the good news: there's hope! Research shows that a healthy, low-purine diet can significantly reduce gout flare-ups and improve your overall health. In fact, some dietary changes that benefit gout also reduce the risk of heart disease, obesity, and even certain cancers – all concerns that become more important as we age. This isn't about deprivation; it's about unlocking a world of delicious, gout-friendly meals that empower you to take control of your health and live a vibrant life. Imagine waking up pain-free, ready to spend your day gardening, golfing, or simply enjoying time with loved ones.

That's where *The Complete Gout-Friendly Cookbook for Seniors comes* in. This book is your one-stop guide to sound nutrition science, packed with simple, delicious recipes designed specifically for seniors with gout. The recipes are easy to follow, can be prepared in a short amount of time, and prioritize fresh, readily available ingredients that are gentle on your joints. You'll spend less time struggling in the kitchen and more time doing the things you love, pain-free.

The Complete Gout-Friendly Cookbook for Seniors will help you navigate the world of healthy eating for gout. We'll explore which foods are truly "gout-friendly" and which to limit in your diet. You'll gain a clear understanding of uric acid and how to control your levels, discovering which purine-containing foods are best avoided and which can be enjoyed in moderation.

This cookbook is more than just a collection of recipes; it's a roadmap to a healthier, happier you. Let's get started on your journey to gout management and a life filled with delicious possibilities – a life where you can wake up feeling good and ready to tackle the day, pain-free!

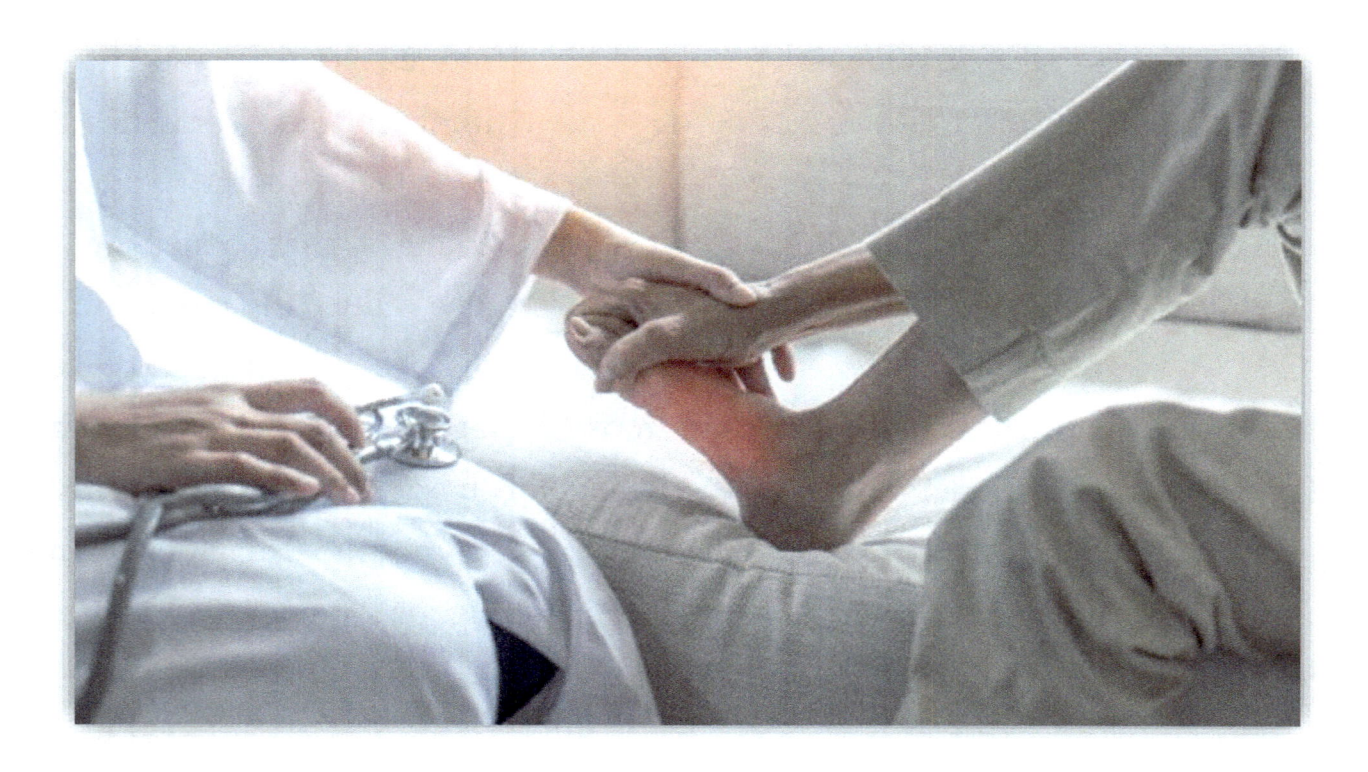

Chapter 1: Understanding Gout in Older Adults

1.1 What is Gout

Gout is a type of inflammatory arthritis that is particularly prevalent among older adults. It is caused by the buildup of uric acid crystals in the joints, leading to sudden, severe joint pain, often starting in the big toe. This condition can be very disruptive to the daily lives of seniors, making it difficult to perform even the most basic tasks.

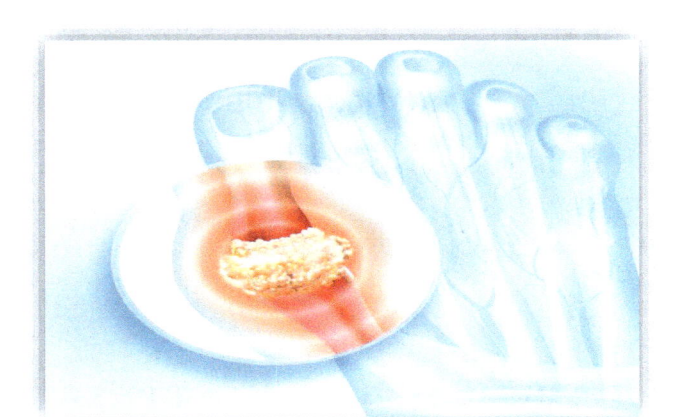

Imagine your bones as a strong and supportive structure. Inside, they resemble a honeycomb. This honeycomb is made of calcium and other minerals, which give bones their strength and rigidity. Think of these minerals as the building blocks that hold the honeycomb together. In between the hard honeycomb sections are softer areas filled with a spongy material called bone marrow. This marrow acts like a factory, constantly producing new blood cells that keep your body functioning properly.

The primary symptom of gout is a sudden, intense pain in the affected joint, accompanied by swelling, redness, and tenderness. These symptoms can make it challenging for older adults to move the joint, which can be especially problematic for those who rely on their mobility to maintain their independence. Additionally, the pain associated with gout attacks can be so severe that it can disrupt sleep and daily routines, further impacting the quality of life for seniors.

It's important to note that gout attacks can come and go, with periods of relief in between. However, this condition should not be ignored, as it can lead to more serious complications if left untreated.

1.2 How Gout Attacks Develop

The underlying cause of gout is the buildup of uric acid crystals in the joints. When uric acid levels in the blood become too high (a condition known as *hyperuricemia*), these crystals can form and accumulate in the joints, triggering an inflammatory response and the characteristic symptoms of gout.

In older adults, there are several factors that can contribute to the development of *hyperuricemia* and, consequently, gout attacks. These include:

- **Diet high in purine-rich foods**: Purines are compounds that can be broken down into uric acid, and foods such as red meat, seafood, and alcohol are particularly high in purines. Studies have shown that higher levels of seafood and meat consumption are associated with a higher risk of gout in the elderly.
- **Dehydration**: Inadequate fluid intake can lead to a decrease in the body's ability to flush out excess uric acid, increasing the risk of crystal formation. Dehydration is a common issue among seniors, especially those living in long-term care facilities.
- **Certain medications**: Diuretics and aspirin, which are commonly prescribed to older adults, can interfere with the body's ability to excrete uric acid, leading to its buildup. A study found that the use of diuretics was associated with a 2.98- to 59.33-fold increased risk of developing gout before age 65.

Gout attacks often occur at night or in the early morning hours, when uric acid levels in the body are typically highest. This can be especially disruptive for seniors, as it can disrupt their sleep and make it difficult to start their day. In fact, a study found that the crude incidence rates of dementia were significantly higher in older adults with gout compared to those without (17.9 vs. 10.9 per 1,000 person-years).

1.3. Risk Factors for Gout

Older adults, particularly those with certain medical conditions or lifestyle factors, should be regularly screened for gout. This is because the risk of developing gout increases significantly with age, and early detection and management can help prevent painful gout attacks and long-term complications. Here are key factors;

- **Obesity and Metabolic Conditions**

Seniors who are overweight or obese are at a higher risk of developing gout. This is because excess body weight can lead to higher levels of uric acid in the blood, which can then crystallize and accumulate in the joints. Conditions like metabolic syndrome, which involve a combination of obesity, high blood pressure, and high cholesterol, also increase the risk of gout in older adults.

- **Kidney Disease**

As we age, our kidneys may not function as efficiently as they once did. This can make it harder for the body to remove excess uric acid, leading to its buildup and the development of gout. Seniors with kidney disease, including chronic kidney disease, are particularly susceptible to gout.

- **Genetics and Family History**

Certain genetic factors can predispose individuals to developing gout. If you have a close family member with gout, you may be at a higher risk of developing the condition as you get older.

- **Certain Medical Conditions**

Conditions like high blood pressure, diabetes, and heart disease, which are more common in the elderly, have also been linked to an increased risk of gout. These conditions can contribute to the buildup of uric acid in the body.

When it comes to the differences in gout risk between senior women and senior men, the data shows that gout is more prevalent in men. In fact, the prevalence of gout is 2 to 6 times higher in men compared to women of the same age. This is likely due to the protective effect of estrogen in women, which helps to regulate uric acid levels in the body.

Understanding gout is crucial for older adults as they are at a higher risk of developing this painful condition. By recognizing the symptoms, risk factors, and impact of gout on daily life, you can take proactive steps to manage and prevent gout attacks. Regular screening for gout, especially for those with obesity, kidney disease, a family history of gout, or certain medical conditions, can help in early detection and effective management.

Moving forward to Chapter 2 on the Diagnosis and Treatment of Gout, we will discuss the essential steps involved in diagnosing gout, including blood tests, joint fluid analysis, and imaging studies. We will also explore the various treatment options available for managing gout, such as lifestyle modifications, medications, and preventive strategies. By understanding how gout is diagnosed and treated, you can work with your healthcare providers to effectively manage this condition and improve your quality of life.

Chapter 2: Diagnosis and Treatment of Gout

2.1 Diagnostic tests for gout

Accurately diagnosing gout is essential for providing appropriate treatment and managing the condition effectively. Healthcare providers typically rely on a combination of different diagnostic tests to confirm the presence of gout in their patients, especially older adults who may be at a higher risk of developing this form of arthritis.

Joint Fluid Analysis

The gold standard for diagnosing gout is the examination of joint fluid under a microscope. This procedure, known as a joint fluid test or *arthrocentesis*, involves the healthcare provider using a small needle to extract a sample of fluid from the affected joint, typically the big toe, knee, or ankle.

The joint fluid sample is then analyzed for the presence of urate crystals, which are the hallmark of gout. These needle-shaped crystals, when viewed under a microscope, have a distinctive appearance that helps differentiate gout from other types of arthritis. The identification of these urate crystals in the joint fluid provides a definitive diagnosis of gout.

Blood Tests

In addition to the joint fluid test, healthcare providers may also order blood tests to measure the levels of uric acid in the patient's bloodstream. Elevated uric acid levels, a condition known as hyperuricemia, are a key indicator of gout.

However, it's important to note that high uric acid levels alone do not necessarily mean that a person has gout. Some individuals may have high uric acid levels without ever developing the painful symptoms of gout. Conversely, some people with gout may have normal or even low uric acid levels during a flare-up.

Therefore, while blood tests can provide valuable information, they should be interpreted in conjunction with the patient's symptoms and the results of the joint fluid analysis to confirm a gout diagnosis.

Imaging Tests

Healthcare providers may also utilize various imaging techniques to support the diagnosis of gout and rule out other potential causes of joint pain and inflammation.

- X-rays: These imaging tests can help identify the presence of urate crystal deposits in the affected joints, as well as any joint damage or changes that may have occurred due to gout.
- Ultrasound: This non-invasive imaging technique can detect the presence of urate crystals in the joints and surrounding tissues, as well as any inflammation or joint damage.
- Dual-energy CT scans: This advanced imaging method can provide detailed images of the joints and accurately identify the presence of urate crystals, even in the early stages of gout.

By combining the results of joint fluid analysis, blood tests, and imaging studies, healthcare providers can arrive at a comprehensive and accurate diagnosis of gout, which is essential for developing an effective treatment plan for older adults.

2.2 Conventional treatment options for gout

The management of gout often involves a combination of pharmacological interventions to address both the acute symptoms of gout attacks and the long-term prevention of future flare-ups. These conventional treatment options play a crucial role in helping individuals, especially older adults, effectively control their gout and minimize the impact on their quality of life.

Medications for Acute Gout Attacks

Non-Steroidal Anti-Inflammatory Drugs **(NSAIDs):** NSAIDs are a common first-line treatment for managing the intense pain and inflammation associated with acute gout attacks. Medications like ibuprofen (Advil, Motrin) and naproxen (Aleve) work by inhibiting the production of inflammatory substances, providing relief during the initial stages of a gout flare-up. These over-the-counter medications can be effective in treating mild to moderate gout attacks, but they should be used with caution in older adults, as they can increase the risk of gastrointestinal bleeding, kidney problems, and cardiovascular events.

Colchicine: Colchicine is a unique anti-inflammatory medication that specifically targets the inflammatory response triggered by the buildup of uric acid crystals in the joints. This drug can be used to both treat acute gout attacks and prevent future flare-ups. Colchicine works by disrupting the movement and function of white blood cells, which play a key role in the inflammatory process. While effective, colchicine can cause gastrointestinal side effects, such as nausea, vomiting, and diarrhea, particularly in older adults.

Corticosteroids: In cases where NSAIDs or colchicine are not suitable or effective, healthcare providers may prescribe corticosteroid medications, such as prednisone, to manage acute gout attacks. Corticosteroids are potent anti-inflammatory agents that can quickly reduce swelling, redness, and pain in the affected joints. These medications can be taken orally or injected directly into the joint. However, long-term use of corticosteroids can lead to side effects, including weight gain, high blood pressure, and an increased risk of infection, which is a particular concern for older adults.

2.3 Medications to Prevent Gout Complications

Uric Acid-Lowering Drugs: To prevent future gout attacks and reduce the risk of long-term complications, healthcare providers may prescribe medications that help lower uric acid levels in the body. Two commonly used uric acid-lowering drugs are allopurinol (Zyloprim) and febuxostat (Uloric). Allopurinol works by inhibiting the enzyme responsible for producing uric acid, while febuxostat helps the body excrete excess uric acid more effectively. These medications are typically taken daily and require close monitoring, as they can interact with other drugs and may need to be adjusted for older adults with kidney problems.

Pegloticase: In cases where other uric acid-lowering medications have been ineffective, healthcare providers may consider prescribing pegloticase, a biologic agent administered through intravenous infusion. Pegloticase works by converting uric acid into a more soluble compound, effectively lowering uric acid levels in the body. This treatment option is typically reserved for individuals with severe, treatment-resistant gout who have not responded to other conventional therapies.

By understanding the various pharmacological treatments available for managing gout, older adults can work closely with their healthcare providers to develop a comprehensive treatment plan that addresses their individual needs, minimizes the risk of side effects, and helps them better control their gout symptoms and prevent future complications.

Chapter 3: The Gout Diet Explained

3.1 The role of purines in gout

Purines are a type of chemical compound that are naturally found in many of the foods you eat. When your body breaks down these purines, it produces a waste product called uric acid.

You see, when you have too much uric acid in your bloodstream, it can form sharp, needle-like crystals that settle in your joints, particularly your big toe. This buildup of uric acid crystals is what causes the intense pain, swelling, and inflammation associated with gout.

Here is a chart that showcases the increased risk of gout in older adults, particularly the differences between senior men and senior women:

Age	Men	Women
65	9.0%	3.3%
75	13.3%	6.2%

This chart clearly illustrates the higher risk of gout in older adults, especially senior men compared to senior women. Understanding these statistics can help older adults and their healthcare providers be more vigilant in monitoring and managing gout as part of their overall health and wellness.

The reason for this gender difference is that women tend to have lower uric acid levels than men, thanks to the protective effects of the hormone estrogen. However, as women age and their estrogen levels decline, their risk of gout increases.

So, by understanding the role that purines play in the development of gout, you can take steps to manage your diet and lower your risk of painful gout attacks as you get older. Stay tuned as we explore which foods are high in purines and how you can adjust your eating habits to better control your uric acid levels.

3.3 Benefits of following a gout diet

Adopting a gout-friendly diet can provide significant benefits for both senior men and women in managing this painful condition. Here's why a gout diet is so important:

- **Lowering Uric Acid Levels**

The primary goal of a gout diet is to help lower uric acid levels in the blood. By limiting the intake of high-purine foods, such as red meat, organ meats, and certain seafood, seniors can reduce the amount of uric acid their bodies produce. This, in turn, decreases the risk of urate crystal formation and painful gout flare-ups.

- **Reducing Gout Attack Frequency**

Research shows that following a gout diet can help lower the frequency and severity of gout attacks. This is particularly beneficial for older adults, as gout attacks can be debilitating and disrupt their daily activities. By managing uric acid levels through diet, seniors can experience fewer painful episodes and maintain a better quality of life.

- **Promoting Weight Management**

Maintaining a healthy weight is crucial for seniors with gout. Excess weight, especially around the midsection, can contribute to higher uric acid levels and increase the risk of gout. A gout-friendly diet that emphasizes nutrient-dense, low-purine foods can help seniors achieve and maintain a healthy weight, further reducing their gout symptoms.

- **Improving Overall Health**

A gout diet that focuses on whole, plant-based foods like fruits, vegetables, whole grains, and low-fat dairy can provide additional health benefits for seniors. These nutrient-rich foods can help support cardiovascular health, strengthen the immune system, and prevent other age-related conditions, ultimately enhancing the overall well-being of older adults with gout.

By following a gout diet, both senior men and women can effectively manage their uric acid levels, reduce the frequency and severity of gout attacks, and maintain a healthy weight. This, in turn, can lead to improved mobility, better sleep, and a higher quality of life, empowering older adults to stay active and independent for longer.

3.2 Foods high, moderate, and low in purines

When it comes to managing gout through diet, understanding which foods are high, moderate, and low in purines is essential. Here's a detailed breakdown to help you make informed choices:

High-Purine Foods to Limit or Avoid:

- **Meats**: Organ meats like liver, kidneys, and sweetbreads are high in purines. Other meats such as veal, venison, and duck should also be limited.
- **Seafood**: Anchovies, sardines, herring, mussels, codfish, scallops, trout, tuna, and haddock are seafood options high in purines.
- **Yeast**: Yeast extracts taken as a supplement should be avoided.
- **Gravies and Sauces**: Those made with meat are high in purines and should be limited.
- **Alcohol**: Beer, liquor, and wine (in moderation) can raise uric acid levels and should be limited.

Moderate-Purine Foods to Limit:

- **Meats**: Limit meat and poultry consumption to 4 to 6 ounces per day.
- **Seafood**: Crab, lobster, oysters, and shrimp fall into the moderate-purine category.
- **Vegetables**: Asparagus, cauliflower, spinach, mushrooms, green peas, and beans should be limited to half a cup per day.

- **Grains**: Oats, oatmeal, wheat germ, and bran should be limited in daily consumption.

Low-Purine Foods to Focus On:

- **Low-Fat Dairy**: Include low-fat or fat-free dairy products like milk, cheese, and yogurt in your diet.
- **Fruits and Fruit Juices**: Enjoy a variety of fruits and their juices as part of a low-purine diet.
- **Vegetables**: Non-soy legumes, eggs, and a variety of other vegetables are low in purines and can be consumed freely.
- **Whole Grains**: Opt for whole grains like bread, pasta, rice, and oats as part of a balanced diet.

By focusing on low-purine options like low-fat dairy, fruits, vegetables, and whole grains, you can create a gout-friendly diet that helps manage uric acid levels and reduce the risk of gout attacks. Remember to limit high and moderate-purine foods to maintain a balanced and healthy eating plan.

3.4 Nutritional considerations for seniors with gout

As older adults, seniors face unique nutritional needs and challenges when it comes to managing gout through diet. Here are some important factors to consider:

- **Maintaining a Healthy Weight**

The search results indicate that excess weight is a significant risk factor for gout, particularly in older adults. Helping seniors achieve and maintain a healthy weight through a gout-friendly diet can be crucial in reducing uric acid levels and preventing painful gout attacks.

- **Adequate Protein Intake**

Seniors require a sufficient amount of high-quality protein to maintain muscle mass and overall health. While limiting high-purine meats, it's important for older adults with gout to focus on plant-based protein sources, such as legumes, tofu, and whole grains, to meet their nutritional needs.

- **Micronutrient Considerations**

As people age, they may be at a higher risk of certain micronutrient deficiencies, such as vitamin C, which has been shown to help lower uric acid levels. Ensuring adequate intake of vitamins, minerals, and other essential nutrients through a balanced diet or supplements (if recommended by a healthcare provider) can be beneficial for seniors with gout.

- **Fluid Intake**

Proper hydration is crucial for seniors with gout, as it helps flush out excess uric acid and prevent the formation of crystals in the joints. Encouraging older adults to drink plenty of water and limiting sugary or alcoholic beverages can support gout management.

- **Medication Interactions**

Seniors with gout may be taking various medications, and it's important to be aware of potential interactions between these drugs and certain foods or dietary supplements. Consulting with a healthcare provider or registered dietitian can help seniors navigate these considerations and develop a safe, effective gout management plan.

By addressing these unique nutritional needs and considerations, seniors with gout can better optimize their diet to control uric acid levels, reduce the risk of gout attacks, and maintain overall health and well-being.

3.5 Medication interactions with food

Older adults with gout often take multiple medications, and it's important to be aware of potential interactions between these drugs and certain foods or dietary supplements.

One key interaction to consider is between allopurinol, a common gout medication, and angiotensin-converting enzyme (ACE) inhibitors, which are often prescribed for conditions like high blood pressure. The search results indicate that the concurrent use of allopurinol and ACE inhibitors can increase the risk of severe adverse effects, such as Stevens-Johnson syndrome and blood dyscrasias (abnormal blood cell counts).

Another potential interaction involves colchicine, another gout medication, and statins like simvastatin. The search results note that colchicine can rarely cause myopathy (muscle damage), and when taken with statins, which can also cause myopathy, there is a risk of an additive or synergistic effect. This interaction is more common in seniors who are taking colchicine long-term or at high doses, or those with impaired kidney function.

To manage these medication interactions, the search results recommend that seniors with gout:

- Inform their healthcare providers and pharmacists about all the medications they are taking, including prescriptions, over-the-counter drugs, and supplements.
- Be closely monitored for any signs of adverse effects, such as skin reactions or unexplained fever or sore throat, especially when starting a new medication regimen.
- Report any muscle pain, tenderness, or weakness, particularly if accompanied by malaise or dark urine, as this could be a sign of a statin-colchicine interaction.

By being aware of these potential medication interactions and working closely with their healthcare team, older adults with gout can safely navigate their treatment plan and minimize the risk of adverse effects.

Delicious and Easy Gout-Friendly Recipes for Seniors
Chapter 4: Breakfast Recipes

This breakfast recipes perfectly curated for seniors with gout provides a well-rounded selection of **nutritious** and ***easy-to-prepare*** options. These meals are designed to support overall health and manage uric acid levels, which is crucial for individuals prone to gout flare-ups.

Nutritional Considerations

Each breakfast recipe has been carefully crafted to address the unique dietary needs of older adults. The focus is on incorporating high-quality protein sources, such as eggs, Greek yogurt, and cottage cheese, to help maintain muscle mass and support satiety. Additionally, the recipes emphasize the use of **low-purine** whole grains, fresh fruits, and vegetables, which are essential for managing gout and providing a range of essential vitamins, minerals, and antioxidants.

Ease of Preparation

Recognizing the potential physical limitations of some seniors, the breakfast recipes selected are straightforward and require minimal preparation time. This ensures that older adults can easily incorporate these meals into their daily routines without feeling overwhelmed or fatigued by the cooking process.

Versatility and Customization

Many of the breakfast recipes offer opportunities for personalization and adaptation to individual preferences and dietary requirements. Seniors can adjust ingredient quantities, substitute alternative low-purine options, or incorporate their favorite flavors to create a truly customized dining experience.

Promoting Healthy Habits

By providing a diverse range of gout-friendly breakfast choices, seniors can establish healthier eating patterns and develop a positive relationship with food.

These recipes encourage the consumption of nutrient-dense foods, which can have a profound impact on overall well-being, energy levels, and the management of gout symptoms.

Incorporating these breakfast recipes into a senior's daily routine can contribute to a comprehensive gout management plan, helping to maintain optimal health and quality of life

Greek Yogurt with Fresh Fruit, Chia Seeds, & Almonds

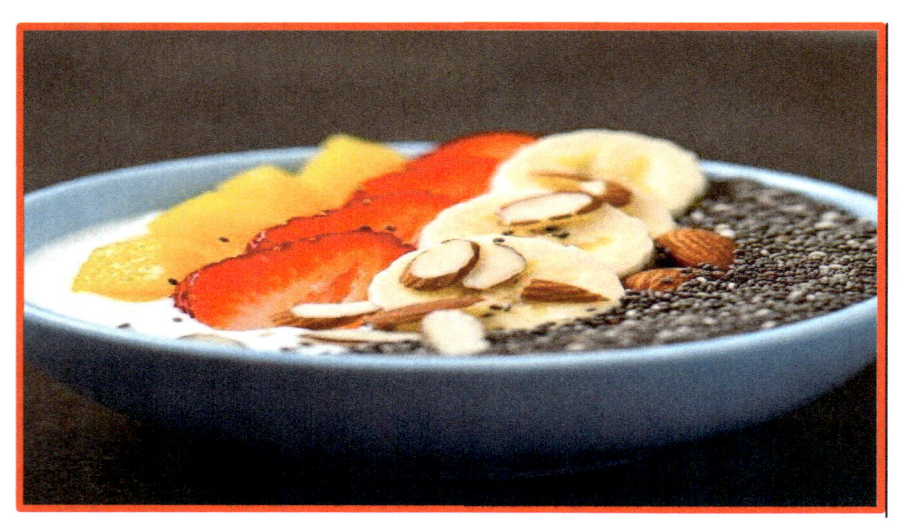

Time of Prep: 10 minutes
Cook Time: None
Serving Size: 1 serving

Nutritional Information (per serving):
- Calories: 250
- Protein: 20g
- Fat: 10g
- Carbohydrates: 20g

Ingredients:
- 1 cup plain Greek yogurt
- 1/2 cup mixed fresh berries (such as blueberries, raspberries, and strawberries)
- 1 tbsp chia seeds
- 1 tbsp sliced almonds

Instructions:
1. In a bowl, combine the Greek yogurt, fresh berries, chia seeds, and sliced almonds.
2. Stir gently to combine.
3. Enjoy immediately or refrigerate until ready to serve.

Avocado Toast with Tomato, Basil, and Smoked Salmon

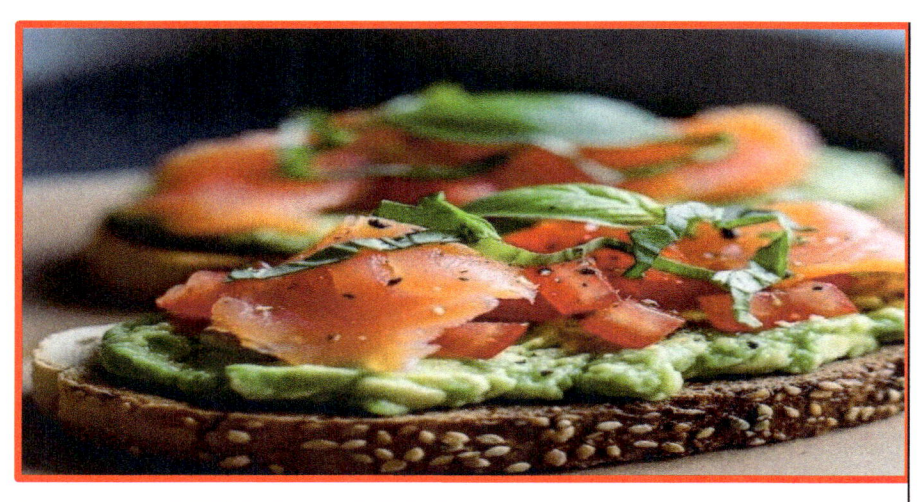

Time of Prep: 10 minutes
Cook Time: None
Serving Size: 1 serving

Nutritional Information (per serving):
- Calories: 300
- Protein: 18g
- Fat: 15g
- Carbohydrates: 25g

Ingredients:
- 2 slices whole grain bread
- 1/2 avocado, mashed
- 1 tomato, diced
- 2-3 fresh basil leaves, chopped
- 2 oz smoked salmon
- Pinch of salt and pepper

Instructions:
1. Toast the whole grain bread until lightly golden.
2. Spread the mashed avocado evenly over the toast slices.
3. Top with diced tomatoes, chopped fresh basil, and smoked salmon.
4. Season with a pinch of salt and pepper.
5. Serve immediately.

Grapefruit and Cottage Cheese with Mixed Nuts

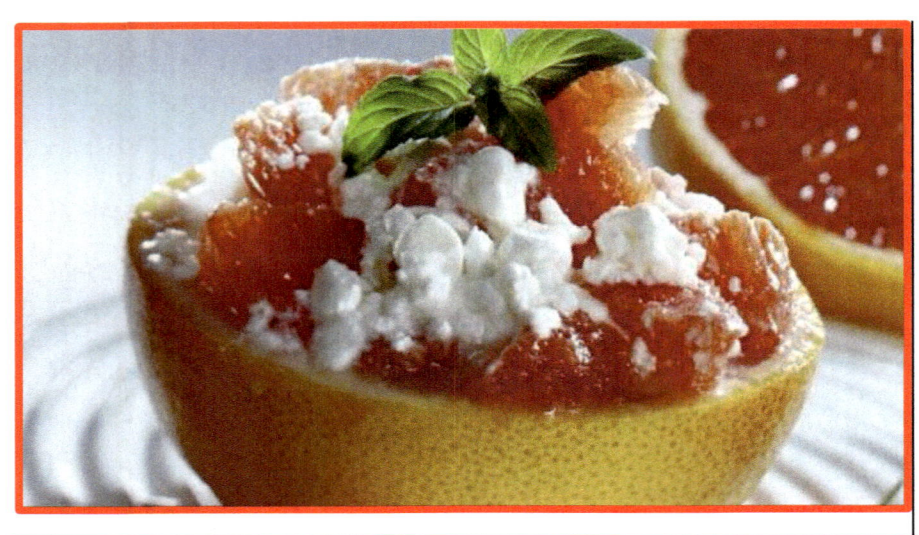

Time of Prep: 5 minutes
Cook Time: None
Serving Size: 1 serving

Nutritional Information (per serving):

- Calories: 200
- Protein: 15g
- Fat: 8g
- Carbohydrates: 20g

Ingredients:

- 1/2 grapefruit, segmented
- 1/2 cup low-fat cottage cheese
- 1 tbsp mixed nuts (such as almonds, walnuts, and pistachios)

Instructions:

1. Segment the grapefruit by cutting along the membranes to release the individual sections.

2. Place the grapefruit segments in a bowl.

3. Top with the low-fat cottage cheese and mixed nuts.

4. Serve immediately.

Whole Wheat Toast with Natural Peanut Butter, Banana, and Chia Seeds

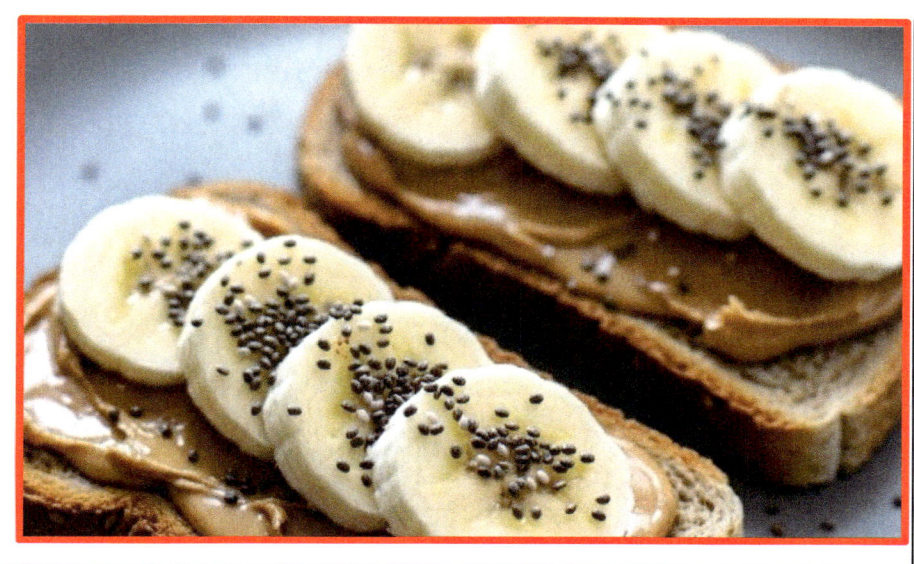

Time of Prep: 5 minutes
Cook Time: None
Serving Size: 1 serving

Nutritional Information (per serving):

- Calories: 320
- Protein: 14g
- Fat: 16g
- Carbohydrates: 37g

Ingredients:

- 2 slices whole wheat bread
- 2 tbsp natural peanut butter (without added sugars or oils)
- 1 small banana, sliced
- 1 tsp chia seeds

Instructions:

1. Toast the whole wheat bread until lightly golden.

2. Spread the natural peanut butter evenly over the toast slices.

3. Top with sliced banana and sprinkle the chia seeds over the top.

4. Serve immediately.

Spinach and Feta Stuffed Mushrooms with Quinoa

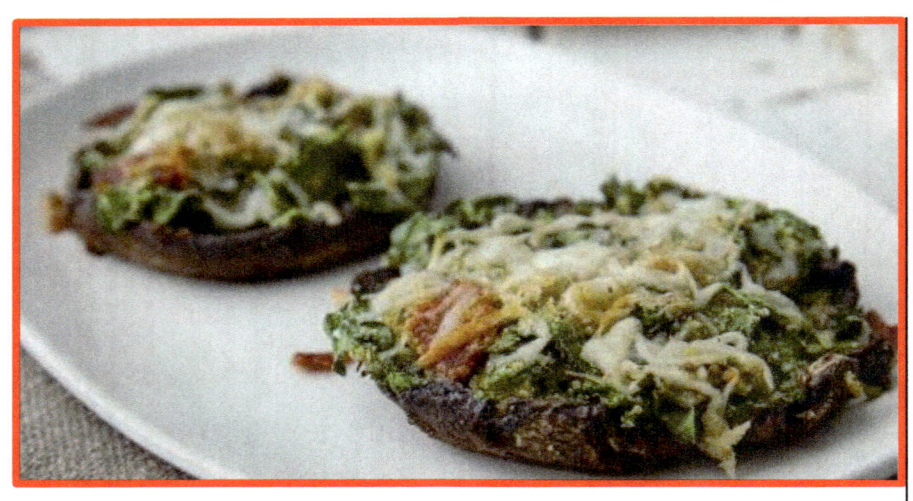

Time of Prep: 15 minutes
Cook Time: 20 minutes
Serving Size: 4 servings

Nutritional Information (per serving):

- Calories: 100
- Protein: 7g
- Fat: 6g
- Carbohydrates: 6g

Ingredients:

- 12 medium-sized mushrooms, stems removed and chopped
- 1 cup fresh spinach, chopped
- 2 oz crumbled feta cheese
- 1/4 cup cooked quinoa
- 1 tbsp olive oil
- 1 garlic clove, minced
- Salt and pepper to taste

Instructions:

1. Preheat the oven to 375°F (190°C).
2. In a skillet, heat the olive oil over medium heat. Add the chopped mushroom stems and garlic. Sauté for 2-3 minutes until fragrant.
3. Add the chopped spinach and sauté until wilted, about 2 minutes.
4. Remove the skillet from heat and stir in the crumbled feta cheese and cooked quinoa. Season with salt and pepper.
5. Stuff the mushroom caps with the spinach-feta-quinoa mixture.
6. Place the stuffed mushrooms on a baking sheet and bake for 15-20 minutes, or until the mushrooms are tender and the filling is heated through.
7. Serve warm.

Baked Oatmeal with Blueberries, Almonds, and Greek Yogurt

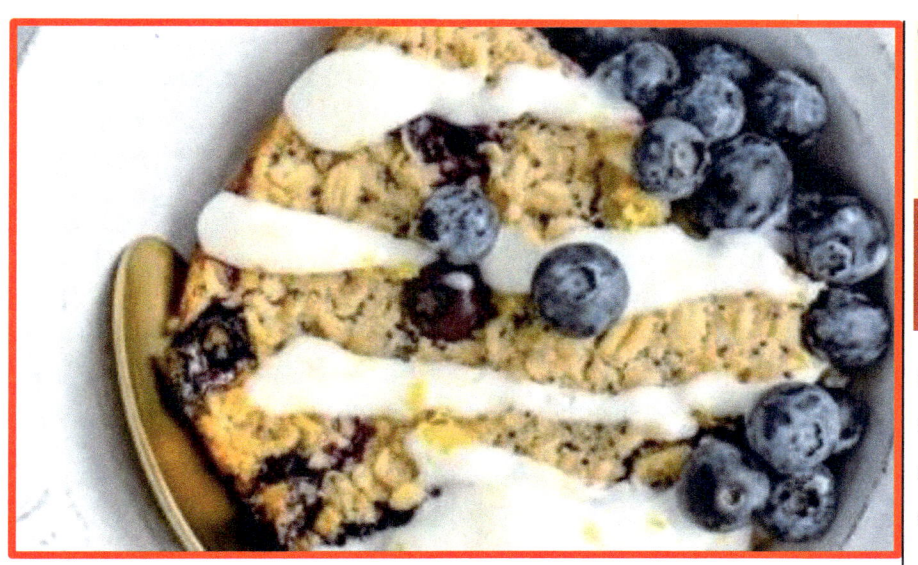

Time of Prep: 10 minutes
Cook Time: 30 minutes
Serving Size: 4 servings

Nutritional Information (per serving):

- Calories: 320
- Protein: 12g
- Fat: 10g
- Carbohydrates: 45g

Ingredients:

- 2 cups old-fashioned oats
- 1 tsp baking powder
- 1/2 tsp ground cinnamon
- 1/4 tsp salt
- 1 cup unsweetened almond milk
- 1/4 cup maple syrup
- 1 egg, lightly beaten
- 1 tsp vanilla extract
- 1 cup fresh or frozen blueberries
- 1/4 cup sliced almonds
- 1/2 cup plain Greek yogurt (for serving)

Instructions:

1. Preheat the oven to 375°F (190°C). Grease an 8x8-inch baking dish.
2. In a large bowl, combine the oats, baking powder, cinnamon, and salt.
3. In a separate bowl, whisk together the almond milk, maple syrup, egg, and vanilla extract.
4. Pour the wet ingredients into the dry ingredients and stir until well combined.
5. Gently fold in the blueberries.
6. Transfer the mixture to the prepared baking dish and top with the sliced almonds.
7. Bake for 25-30 minutes, or until the oatmeal is set and the top is lightly golden.
8. Serve warm, topped with a dollop of plain Greek yogurt.

Veggie Omelet with Goat Cheese and Fresh Herbs

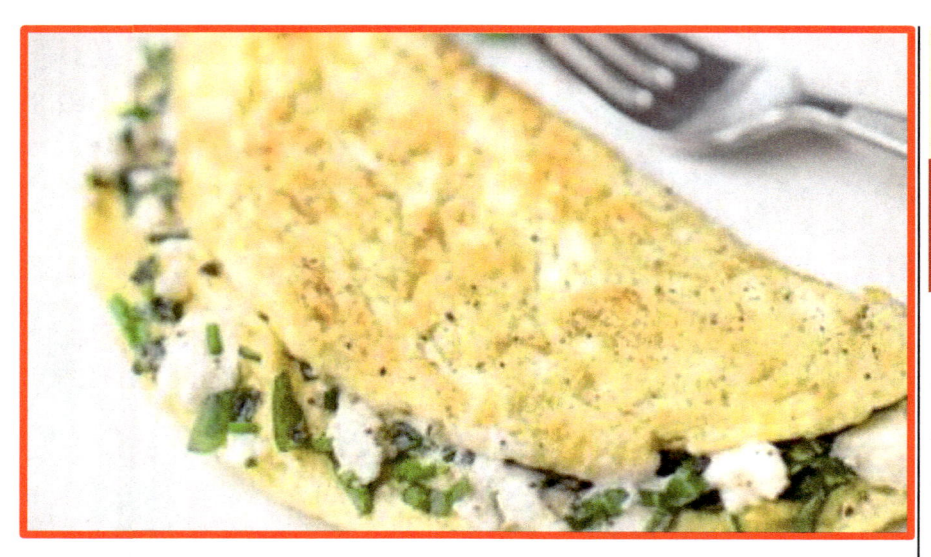

Time of Prep: 15 minutes
Cook Time: 10 minutes
Serving Size: 1 serving

Nutritional Information (per serving):

- Calories: 280
- Protein: 20g
- Fat: 18g
- Carbohydrates: 10g

Ingredients:

- 2 eggs
- 1 tbsp olive oil
- 1/4 cup diced bell pepper
- 1/4 cup diced onion
- 1/4 cup sliced mushrooms
- 1/4 cup baby spinach leaves
- 2 tbsp crumbled goat cheese
- 1 tbsp chopped fresh herbs (such as parsley, dill, or chives)
- Salt and pepper to taste

Instructions:

1. In a small bowl, whisk the eggs and season with a pinch of salt and pepper.
2. Heat the olive oil in a non-stick skillet over medium heat.
3. Add the diced bell pepper, onion, and sliced mushrooms to the skillet. Sauté for 3-4 minutes until the vegetables are tender.
4. Add the baby spinach leaves and sauté until wilted, about 1 minute.
5. Pour the whisked eggs into the skillet and let them cook for 2-3 minutes, or until the bottom is set.
6. Gently fold the omelet in half and sprinkle the crumbled goat cheese and chopped fresh herbs over the top.
7. Cook for an additional 2-3 minutes, or until the cheese is melted and the omelet is cooked through.
8. Slide the omelet onto a plate and serve immediately.

Overnight Oats with Berries, Walnuts, and Protein Powder

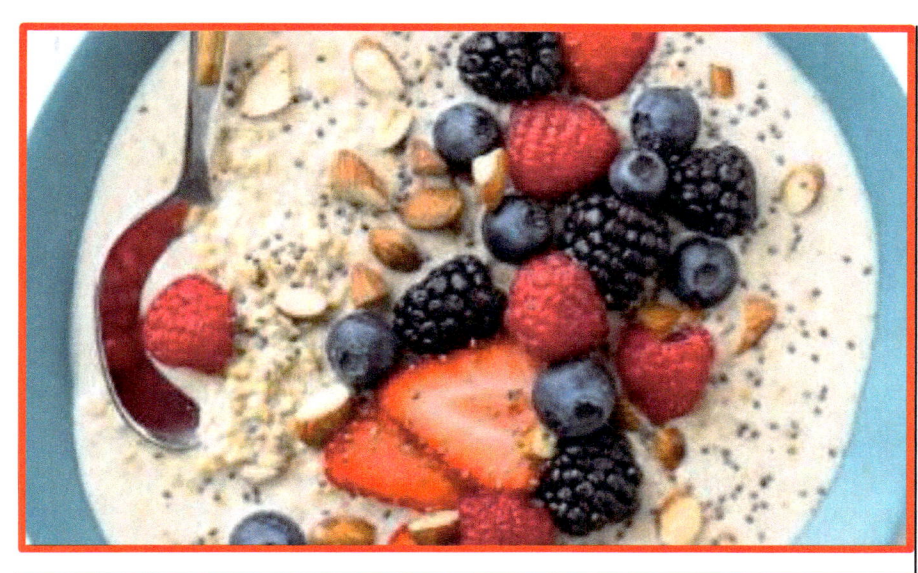

Time of Prep: 5 minutes
Cook Time: None (Overnight)
Serving Size: 1 serving

Nutritional Information (per serving):

- Calories: 380
- Protein: 20g
- Fat: 16g
- Carbohydrates: 42g

Ingredients:

- 1/2 cup steel-cut oats
- 1 cup unsweetened almond milk
- 1 tbsp chia seeds
- 1 tsp honey (optional)
- 1/2 cup mixed berries (such as blueberries, raspberries, and blackberries)
- 2 tbsp chopped walnuts
- 1 scoop vanilla protein powder

Instructions:

1. In a mason jar or airtight container, combine the steel-cut oats, almond milk, chia seeds, and honey (if using).

2. Stir to mix well.

3. Cover and refrigerate overnight or for at least 4 hours.

4. In the morning, top the overnight oats with the mixed berries, chopped walnuts, and a scoop of vanilla protein powder.

5. Stir to combine and serve chilled.

Quinoa Porridge with Cinnamon, Apples, and Flaxseed

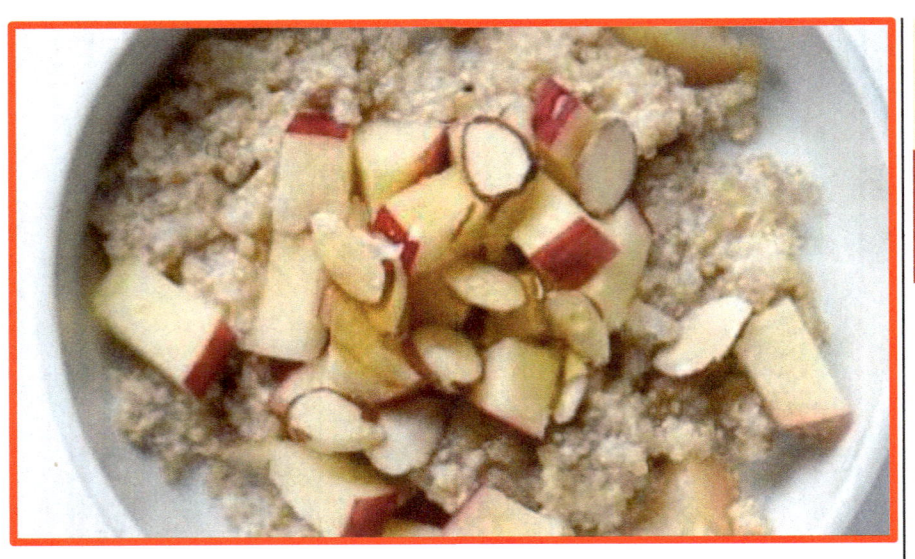

Time of Prep: 10 minutes
Cook Time: 15 minutes
Serving Size: 1 serving

Nutritional Information (per serving):

- Calories: 280
- Protein: 10g
- Fat: 10g
- Carbohydrates: 38g

Ingredients:

- 1/2 cup quinoa, rinsed
- 1 cup unsweetened almond milk
- 1/4 tsp ground cinnamon
- 1 small apple, diced
- 1 tbsp chopped walnuts
- 1 tbsp ground flaxseed

Instructions:

1. In a small saucepan, combine the rinsed quinoa and almond milk.

2. Bring the mixture to a boil over medium heat, then reduce the heat to low and simmer for 12-15 minutes, stirring occasionally, until the quinoa is cooked and the porridge has thickened.

3. Remove the saucepan from heat and stir in the ground cinnamon.

4. Top the quinoa porridge with the diced apple, chopped walnuts, and ground flaxseed.

5. Serve warm.

Egg White Veggie Frittata with Kale and Fresh Herbs

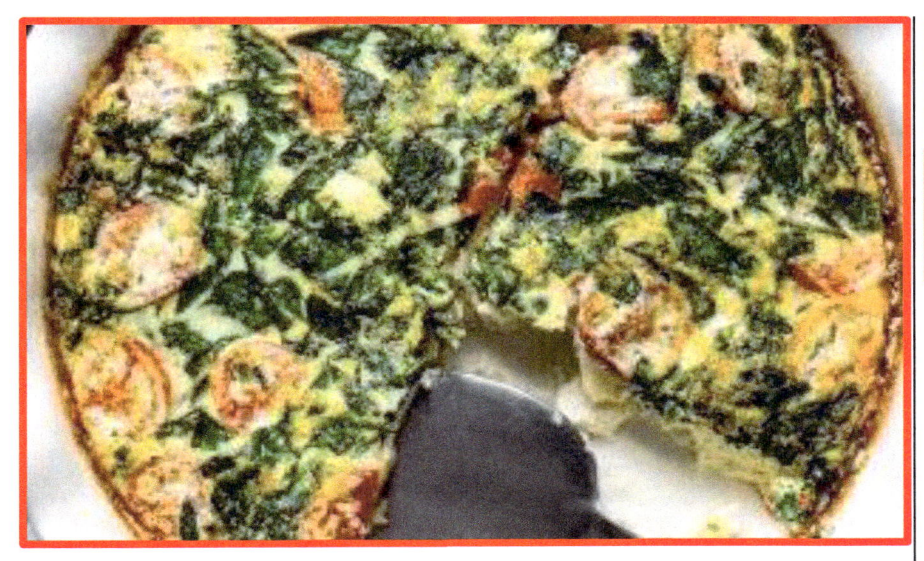

Time of Prep: 15 minutes
Cook Time: 20 minutes
Serving Size: 4 servings

Nutritional Information (per serving):

- Calories: 110
- Protein: 14g
- Fat: 4g
- Carbohydrates: 6g

Ingredients:

- 6 egg whites
- 1/4 cup diced bell pepper
- 1/4 cup diced onion
- 1/4 cup sliced mushrooms
- 1 cup chopped kale
- 2 tbsp grated low-fat cheddar cheese
- 2 tbsp chopped fresh herbs (such as parsley, basil, or chives)
- Salt and pepper to taste
- Cooking spray

Instructions:

1. Preheat the oven to 375°F (190°C).

2. In a medium bowl, whisk the egg whites and season with a pinch of salt and pepper.

3. Coat a 9-inch oven-safe non-stick skillet with cooking spray and place it over medium heat.

4. Add the diced bell pepper, onion, and sliced mushrooms to the skillet. Sauté for 3-4 minutes until the vegetables are tender.

5. Add the chopped kale and sauté for an additional 1-2 minutes until the kale is wilted.

6. Pour the whisked egg whites into the skillet, making sure to evenly distribute the vegetables and kale.

7. Sprinkle the grated cheddar cheese and chopped fresh herbs over the top.

8. Transfer the skillet to the preheated oven and bake for 15-20 minutes, or until the frittata is set and the cheese is melted.

9. Remove the frittata from the oven and let it cool for a few minutes before slicing and serving.

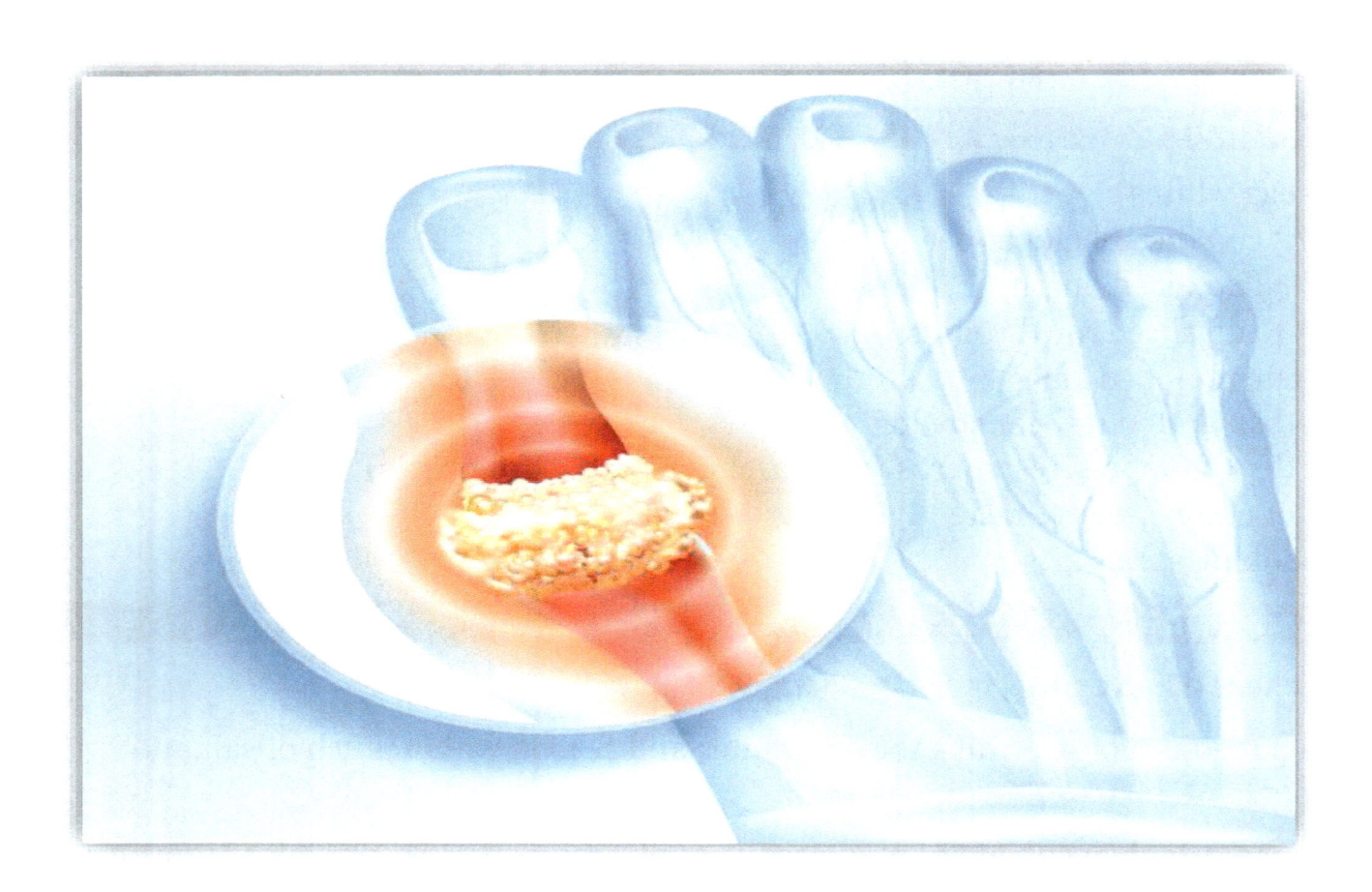

Chapter 5: Lunch Recipes (Light and satisfying meals)

Maintaining a balanced and nutritious diet is crucial for seniors, especially those managing gout. The lunch recipes curated here prioritize simplicity, ease of preparation, and a focus on ingredients that can help manage uric acid levels and support overall health.

These lunch options are designed to be quick and straightforward, recognizing the potential physical limitations and time constraints that some older adults may face. Each recipe incorporates a variety of low-purine foods, such as lean proteins, complex carbohydrates, and nutrient-dense vegetables, to provide a well-rounded and satisfying midday meal.

By following these easy-to-prepare lunch recipes, seniors can enjoy flavorful and gout-friendly meals that support their dietary needs and overall well-being. The recipes are adaptable, allowing for personalization and substitutions to cater to individual preferences and dietary requirements.

Dive into the following selection of senior-friendly lunch recipes and discover delicious and nourishing options that can be easily incorporated into your daily routine.

Whole Grain Chicken Spinach Mushroom Flatbread

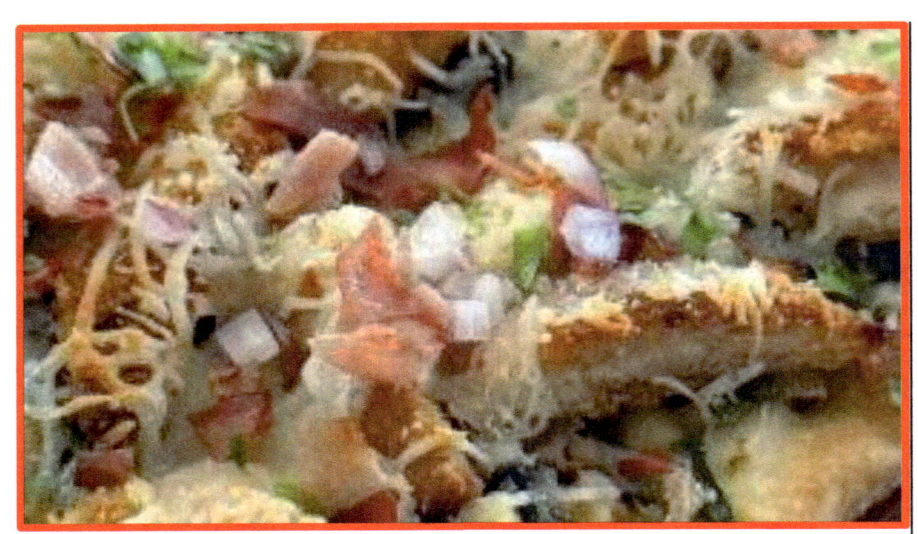

Time of Prep: 20 minutes

Cook Time: 15 minutes

Serving Size: 2 servings

Nutritional Information:

- Calories: 300
- Protein: 25g
- Fat: 12g
- Carbohydrates: 25g

Ingredients:

- 1 whole grain flatbread or naan
- 2 oz cooked, low-sodium chicken breast, shredded
- 1/2 cup sliced mushrooms
- 1 cup fresh spinach leaves
- 2 tbsp crumbled feta cheese
- 1 tbsp olive oil
- Salt and pepper to taste

Instructions:

1. Preheat your oven to 400°F (200°C).
2. Place the whole grain flatbread or naan on a baking sheet.
3. In a small bowl, combine the shredded chicken, sliced mushrooms, and fresh spinach leaves.
4. Spread the chicken-vegetable mixture evenly over the flatbread.
5. Sprinkle the crumbled feta cheese over the top.
6. Drizzle the olive oil over the flatbread and season with a pinch of salt and pepper.
7. Bake in the preheated oven for 12-15 minutes, or until the flatbread is crispy and the cheese is melted.
8. Remove the flatbread from the oven and slice it into desired portions.
9. Serve hot.

Gout Diet for Seniors

Beef & Barley Soup with Leafy Greens

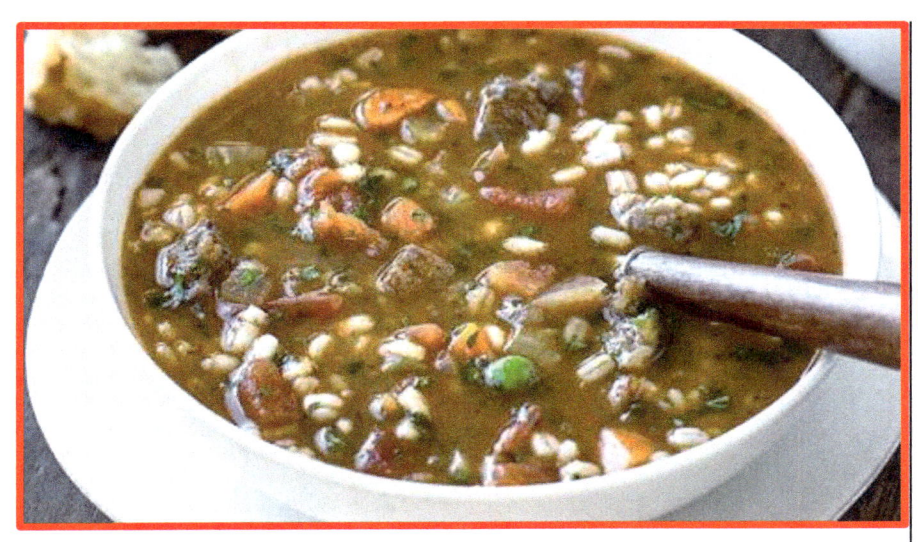

Time of Prep: 20 minutes
Cook Time: 45 minutes
Serving Size: 4 servings

Nutritional Information:

- Calories: 350
- Protein: 30g
- Fat: 10g
- Carbohydrates: 35g

Ingredients:

- 1 lb lean beef stew meat, cubed
- 1 tbsp olive oil
- 1 onion, diced
- 2 carrots, peeled and diced
- 2 celery stalks, diced
- 3 garlic cloves, minced
- 6 cups low-sodium beef broth
- 1 cup pearl barley
- 1 tsp dried thyme
- 2 cups chopped kale or spinach
- Salt and pepper to taste

Instructions:

1. In a large pot or Dutch oven, heat the olive oil over medium-high heat.

2. Add the cubed beef and brown it on all sides, about 5-7 minutes. Remove the beef from the pot and set it aside.

3. Reduce the heat to medium and add the diced onion, carrots, and celery to the pot. Sauté the vegetables for 5-7 minutes, or until they start to soften.

4. Add the minced garlic and sauté for an additional minute, until fragrant.

5. Pour in the low-sodium beef broth and stir in the pearl barley.

6. Return the browned beef to the pot and add the dried thyme.

7. Bring the soup to a boil, then reduce the heat to low, cover, and simmer for 30-40 minutes, or until the barley is tender and the beef is cooked through.

8. Stir in the chopped kale or spinach and cook for an additional 5 minutes, or until the greens are wilted.

9. Season with salt and pepper to taste.

10. Serve hot.

Salad with Cheese, Avocado, and Hard-Boiled Egg

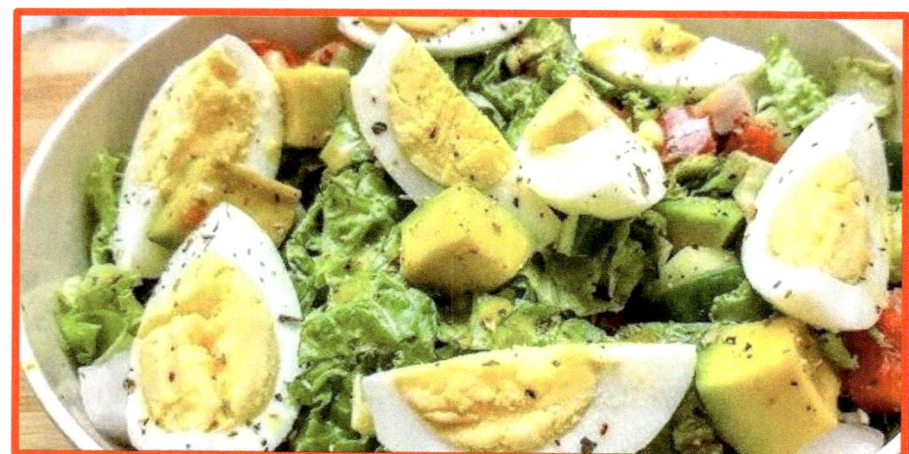

Time of Prep: 15 minutes
Cook Time: None
Serving Size: 1 serving

Nutritional Information (per serving):

- Calories: 400
- Protein: 18g
- Fat: 32g
- Carbohydrates: 16g

Ingredients:

- 2 cups mixed greens (such as spinach, arugula, and kale)
- 1/2 avocado, sliced
- 2 hard-boiled eggs, sliced
- 2 tbsp crumbled feta or goat cheese
- 2 tbsp chopped walnuts
- 2 tbsp olive oil
- 1 tbsp balsamic vinegar
- Salt and pepper to taste

Instructions:

1. In a large salad bowl, combine the mixed greens, sliced avocado, sliced hard-boiled eggs, crumbled cheese, and chopped walnuts.

2. Drizzle the olive oil and balsamic vinegar over the salad and toss gently to coat.

3. Season with salt and pepper to taste.

4. Serve immediately.

Gout Diet for Seniors

Whole Grain Ham and Cheese Panini

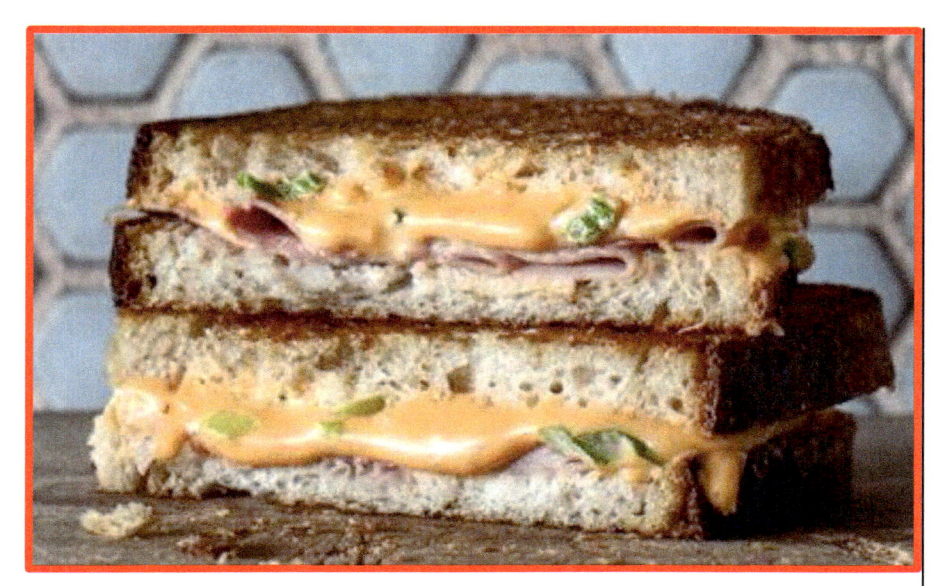

Time of Prep: 10 minutes

Cook Time: 5-7 minutes

Serving Size: 1 serving

Nutritional Information (per serving):

- Calories: 300
- Protein: 22g
- Fat: 12g
- Carbohydrates: 28g

Ingredients:

- 2 slices whole grain bread
- 2 oz low-sodium ham, thinly sliced
- 1 oz low-fat cheddar cheese, sliced
- 1 tsp Dijon mustard
- 1 tsp olive oil

Instructions:

1. Preheat a panini press or grill pan over medium heat.
2. Spread the Dijon mustard on one slice of whole grain bread.
3. Layer the sliced low-sodium ham and low-fat cheddar cheese on the mustard-coated bread.
4. Top with the remaining slice of whole grain bread.
5. Brush the outside of the sandwich with the olive oil.
6. Place the sandwich in the preheated panini press or grill pan and cook for 5-7 minutes, or until the bread is golden brown and the cheese is melted.
7. Remove the sandwich from the heat and slice it in half diagonally.
8. Serve immediately.

Turkey, Avocado, and Tomato Wrap with Spinach

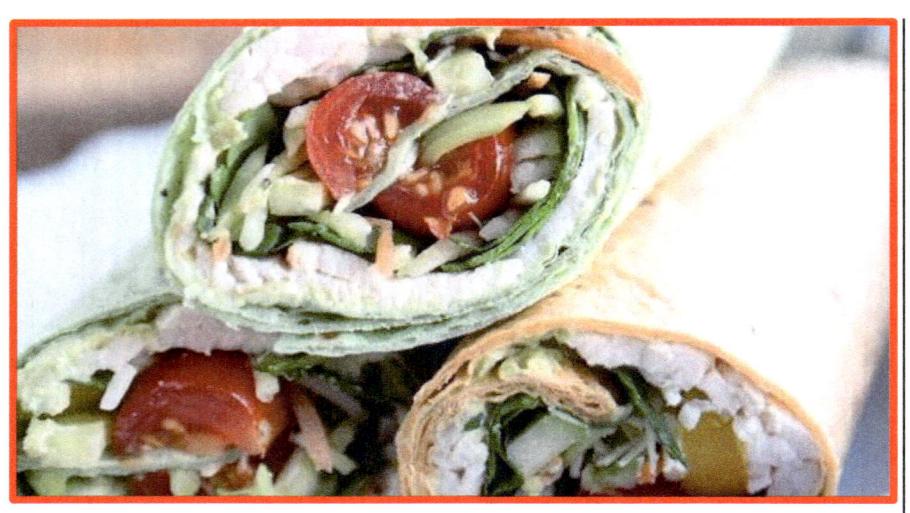

Time of Prep: 10 minutes
Cook Time: None
Serving Size: 1 serving

Nutritional Information (per serving):

- Calories: 350
- Protein: 22g
- Fat: 18g
- Carbohydrates: 28g

Ingredients:

- 1 whole wheat or spinach wrap
- 3 oz sliced turkey breast
- 1/2 avocado, sliced
- 1 tomato, sliced
- 1 cup fresh spinach leaves
- 1 tbsp olive oil
- 1 tbsp balsamic vinegar
- Salt and pepper to taste

Instructions:

1. Lay the whole wheat or spinach wrap on a flat surface.
2. Layer the sliced turkey breast, avocado slices, tomato slices, and fresh spinach leaves in the center of the wrap.
3. Drizzle the olive oil and balsamic vinegar over the filling.
4. Season with salt and pepper to taste.
5. Fold the bottom of the wrap up, then fold in the sides and continue rolling tightly to enclose the filling.
6. Serve immediately.

Vegetable Omelet with Feta Cheese

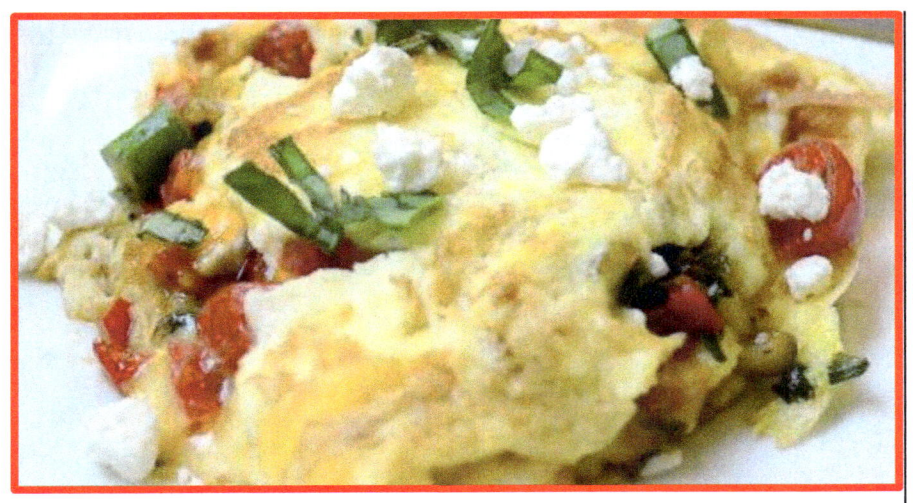

Time of Prep: 15 minutes
Cook Time: 10 minutes
Serving Size: 1 serving

Nutritional Information (per serving):

- Calories: 280
- Protein: 20g
- Fat: 16g
- Carbohydrates: 10g

Ingredients:

- 2 eggs
- 1 tbsp olive oil
- 1/4 cup diced bell pepper
- 1/4 cup diced onion
- 1/4 cup sliced mushrooms
- 1/4 cup chopped tomatoes
- 2 tbsp crumbled feta cheese
- Salt and pepper to taste

Instructions:

1. In a small bowl, whisk the eggs and season with a pinch of salt and pepper.
2. Heat the olive oil in a non-stick skillet over medium heat.
3. Add the diced bell pepper, onion, sliced mushrooms, and chopped tomatoes to the skillet. Sauté for 3-4 minutes until the vegetables are tender.
4. Pour the whisked eggs into the skillet and let them cook for 2-3 minutes, or until the bottom is set.
5. Sprinkle the crumbled feta cheese over the top of the omelet.
6. Gently fold the omelet in half and cook for an additional 2-3 minutes, or until the cheese is melted and the omelet is cooked through.
7. Slide the omelet onto a plate and serve immediately.

Whole Wheat Mac 'n Cheese with Ham and Broccoli

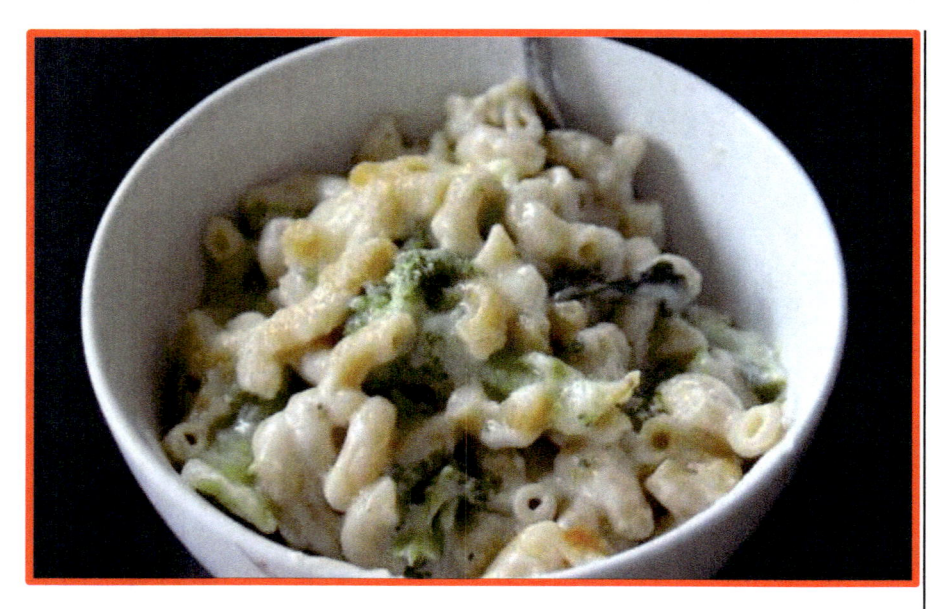

Time of Prep: 20 minutes

Cook Time: 25 minutes

Serving Size: 4 servings

Nutritional Information (per serving):

- Calories: 400
- Protein: 25g
- Fat: 15g
- Carbohydrates: 40g

Ingredients:

- 8 oz whole wheat elbow macaroni
- 2 tbsp olive oil
- 2 tbsp all-purpose flour
- 2 cups low-fat milk
- 1 cup shredded low-fat cheddar cheese
- 1/4 cup grated Parmesan cheese
- 1 tsp Dijon mustard
- 1/4 tsp ground nutmeg
- Salt and pepper to taste
- 4 oz diced ham
- 1 cup steamed broccoli florets

Instructions:

1. Preheat your oven to 375°F (190°C).
2. Cook the whole wheat elbow macaroni according to the package instructions. Drain and set aside.
3. In a medium saucepan, heat the olive oil over medium heat. Whisk in the all-purpose flour and cook for 1-2 minutes, stirring constantly, to create a roux.
4. Gradually whisk in the low-fat milk and bring the mixture to a simmer. Cook, stirring occasionally, until the sauce thickens, about 5-7 minutes.
5. Remove the saucepan from heat and stir in the shredded low-fat cheddar

cheese, grated Parmesan cheese, Dijon mustard, and ground nutmeg. Season with salt and pepper to taste.

6. Add the cooked macaroni, diced ham, and steamed broccoli florets to the cheese sauce and stir to combine.

7. Transfer the mac and cheese mixture to a baking dish and bake in the preheated oven for 20-25 minutes, or until the top is golden brown and bubbly.

8. Remove the mac and cheese from the oven and let it cool for a few minutes before serving.

Roast Chicken with Garlic Potatoes and Glazed Carrots

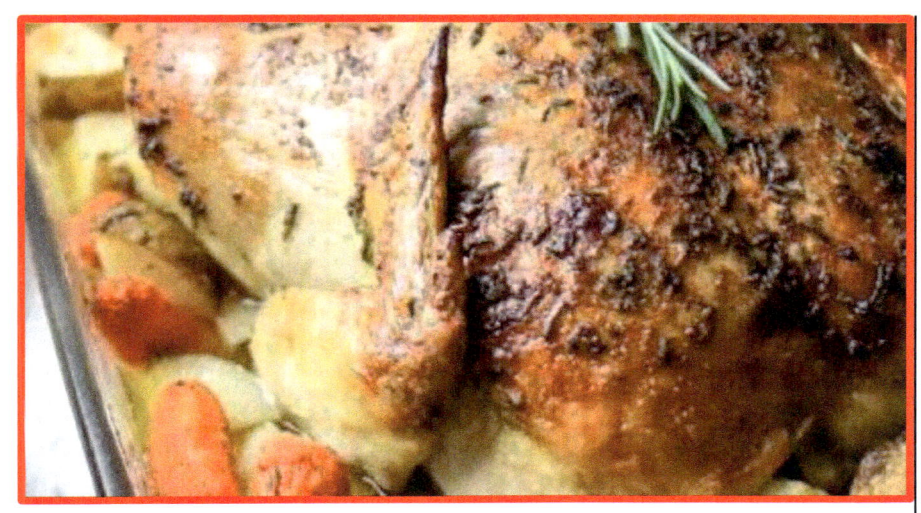

Time of Prep: 20 minutes
Cook Time: 45 minutes
Serving Size: 4 servings

Nutritional Information (per serving):
- Calories: 400
- Protein: 35g
- Fat: 10g
- Carbohydrates: 40g

Ingredients:

- 1 lb boneless, skinless chicken breasts
- lbs red potatoes, cubed
- 4 carrots, peeled and cut into 1-inch pieces
- 2 tbsp olive oil, divided
- 3 garlic cloves, minced
- 1 tsp dried thyme
- Salt and pepper to taste
- 2 tbsp honey

Instructions:

1. Preheat your oven to 400°F (200°C).
2. In a large baking dish, toss the cubed red potatoes with 1 tbsp of olive oil,

minced garlic, dried thyme, and a pinch of salt and pepper.

3. Arrange the potato mixture in an even layer and roast in the preheated oven for 20 minutes.
4. Meanwhile, season the boneless, skinless chicken breasts with salt and pepper.
5. Heat the remaining 1 tbsp of olive oil in a large skillet over medium-high heat. Add the chicken breasts and sear them for 2-3 minutes per side, or until they are lightly browned.
6. Remove the partially roasted potatoes from the oven and add the seared chicken breasts to the baking dish. Return the dish to the oven and continue roasting for an additional 20-25 minutes, or until the chicken is cooked through and the potatoes are tender.
7. In a separate baking dish, toss the peeled and cut carrots with the honey. Roast the carrots in the oven for 15-20 minutes, or until they are tender and glazed.
8. Serve the roast chicken, garlic potatoes, and glazed carrots together.

Baked Salmon with Quinoa and Steamed Broccoli

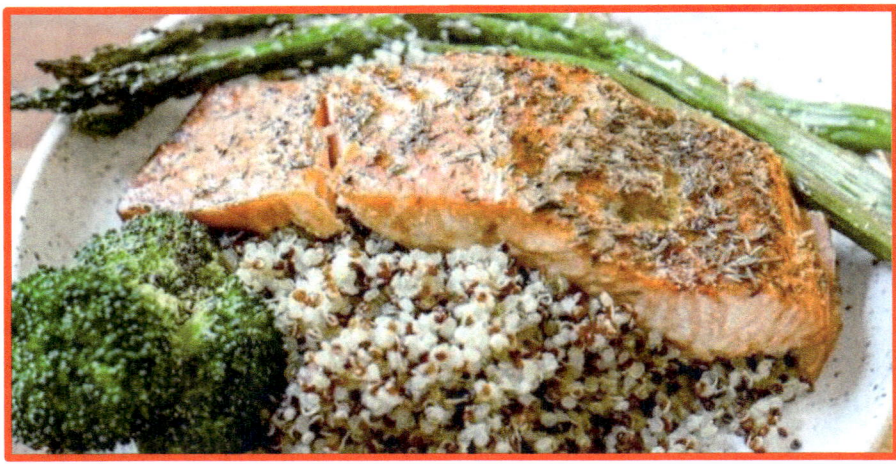

Time of Prep: 15 minutes
Cook Time: 25 minutes
Serving Size: 2 servings

Nutritional Information (per serving):

- Calories: 350
- Protein: 30g
- Fat: 15g
- Carbohydrates: 25g

Ingredients:

- 2 (4 oz) wild-caught salmon fillets
- 1 cup cooked quinoa
- 2 cups broccoli florets
- 1 tbsp olive oil

- 1 tbsp lemon juice
- 1 tsp dried dill
- Salt and pepper to taste

Instructions:

1. Preheat your oven to 400°F (200°C).
2. Place the salmon fillets on a baking sheet lined with parchment paper. Drizzle the fillets with 1 tbsp of olive oil and season with salt, pepper, and dried dill.
3. Bake the salmon in the preheated oven for 15-20 minutes, or until it flakes easily with a fork.
4. While the salmon is baking, steam the broccoli florets until they are tender, about 5-7 minutes.
5. In a small bowl, combine the cooked quinoa, steamed broccoli, 1 tbsp of olive oil, and lemon juice. Season with salt and pepper to taste.
6. Serve the baked salmon fillets alongside the quinoa and broccoli mixture.

Hearty Beef and Root Vegetable Stew

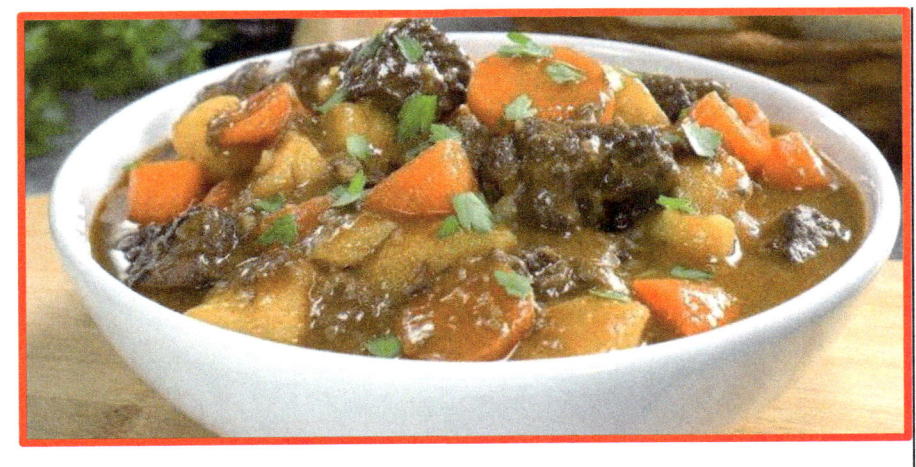

Time of Prep: 20 minutes
Cook Time: 1 hour
Serving Size: 4 servings

Nutritional Information (per serving):
- Calories: 300
- Protein: 25g
- Fat: 10g
- Carbohydrates: 30g

Ingredients:

- 1 lb lean beef stew meat, cubed
- 1 tbsp olive oil
- 1 onion, diced

- 2 carrots, peeled and diced
- 2 parsnips, peeled and diced
- 2 cups low-sodium beef broth
- 1 cup diced tomatoes
- 1 cup chopped butternut squash
- 1 tsp dried rosemary
- Salt and pepper to taste

Instructions:

1. In a large pot or Dutch oven, heat the olive oil over medium-high heat.
2. Add the cubed beef and brown it on all sides, about 5-7 minutes. Remove the beef from the pot and set it aside.
3. Reduce the heat to medium and add the diced onion, carrots, and parsnips to the pot. Sauté the vegetables for 5-7 minutes, or until they start to soften.
4. Add the diced tomatoes, chopped butternut squash, and dried rosemary to the pot.
5. Return the browned beef to the pot and pour in the low-sodium beef broth.
6. Bring the stew to a boil, then reduce the heat to low, cover, and simmer for 45-60 minutes, or until the beef is tender and the vegetables are cooked through.
7. Season with salt and pepper to taste.
8. Serve hot.

Chapter 6: Dinner Recipes (Hearty and flavorful dishes)

Maintaining a balanced and gout-friendly diet is crucial for seniors managing the symptoms of gout. This collection of dinner recipes has been carefully crafted to not only provide delicious and satisfying meals but also to support the overall health and well-being of those living with gout.

The recipes featured in this collection are designed to be low in purines, a key factor in managing gout. By focusing on lean proteins, complex carbohydrates, and a variety of nutrient-dense vegetables, these meals can help reduce the risk of gout flare-ups and promote better joint health. The inclusion of ingredients like salmon, lentils, and whole grains provides essential nutrients that can help alleviate inflammation and support the body's natural defenses against gout.

Marinated Baked Salmon with Herb-Roasted Vegetables

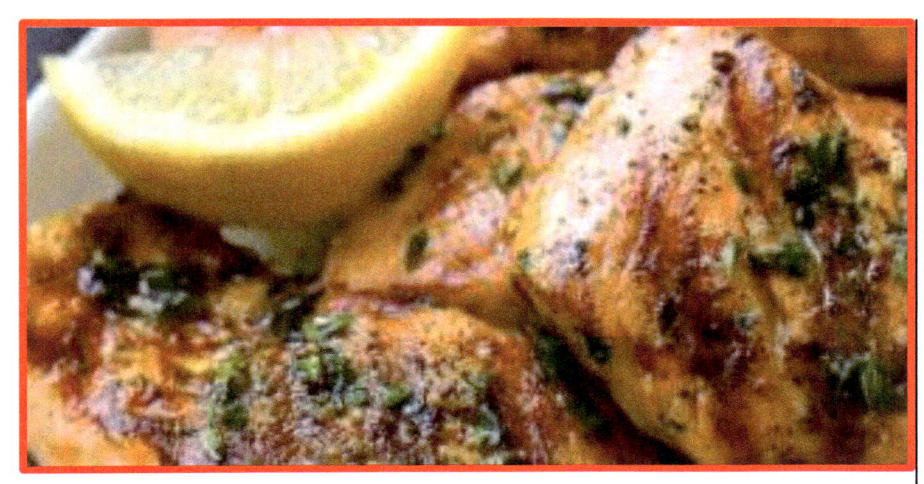

Time of Prep: 20 minutes
Cook Time: 30 minutes
Serving Size: 2 servings

Nutritional Information (per serving):
- Calories: 350
- Protein: 30g
- Fat: 18g
- Carbohydrates: 15g

Ingredients:

- 2 (4 oz) wild-caught salmon fillets
- 2 cups mixed vegetables (such as broccoli, bell peppers, and zucchini), chopped
- 2 tbsp olive oil, divided

- 1 tsp dried dill
- Salt and pepper to taste
- Marinade: Lemon juice, fresh herbs (such as parsley and thyme), olive oil

Instructions:

1. Preheat your oven to 400°F (200°C).
2. Prepare a marinade using lemon juice, fresh herbs, and olive oil. Marinate the salmon fillets for at least 15 minutes.
3. In a large baking dish, toss the chopped vegetables with 1 tbsp of olive oil, salt, and pepper.
4. Roast the vegetables in the preheated oven for 20 minutes, stirring halfway.
5. Place the marinated salmon fillets on a baking sheet lined with parchment paper.
6. Bake the salmon in the oven for 15-20 minutes, or until it flakes easily with a fork.
7. Serve the baked salmon with the herb-roasted vegetables.

Lean Chicken and Broccoli Stir-Fry

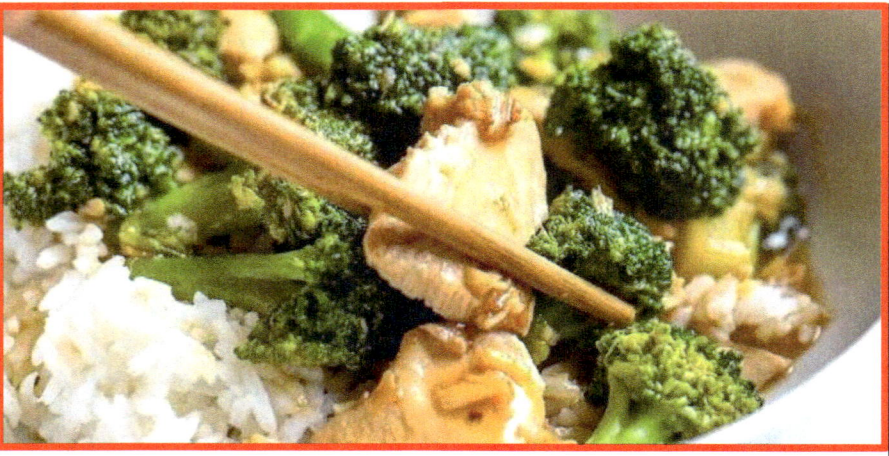

Time of Prep: 15 minutes
Cook Time: 20 minutes
Serving Size: 4 servings

Nutritional Information (per serving):
- Calories: 400
- Protein: 30g
- Fat: 12g
- Carbohydrates: 40g

Ingredients:

- 1 lb lean ground turkey or chicken
- 1 cup cooked quinoa

- 1/2 cup diced onion
- 2 garlic cloves, minced
- 1 tsp dried oregano
- 1/4 tsp red pepper flakes (optional)
- Salt and pepper to taste
- 8 oz whole wheat pasta
- 1 cup low-sodium marinara sauce

Instructions:

1. Preheat your oven to 400°F (200°C).
2. In a large bowl, combine the ground turkey, whole wheat breadcrumbs, beaten egg, grated Parmesan cheese, minced garlic, dried oregano, and red pepper flakes (if using). Mix well and season with salt and pepper.
3. Roll the turkey mixture into 1-inch meatballs and place them on a baking sheet lined with parchment paper.
4. Bake the meatballs in the preheated oven for 20-25 minutes, or until they are cooked through and lightly browned.
5. While the meatballs are baking, cook the whole wheat pasta according to the package instructions. Drain and set aside.
6. In a saucepan, heat the low-sodium marinara sauce over medium heat until warmed through.
7. Add the cooked meatballs to the marinara sauce and stir to coat.
8. Serve the turkey meatballs and sauce over the cooked whole wheat pasta.

Flavorful Lentil and Sweet Potato Curry

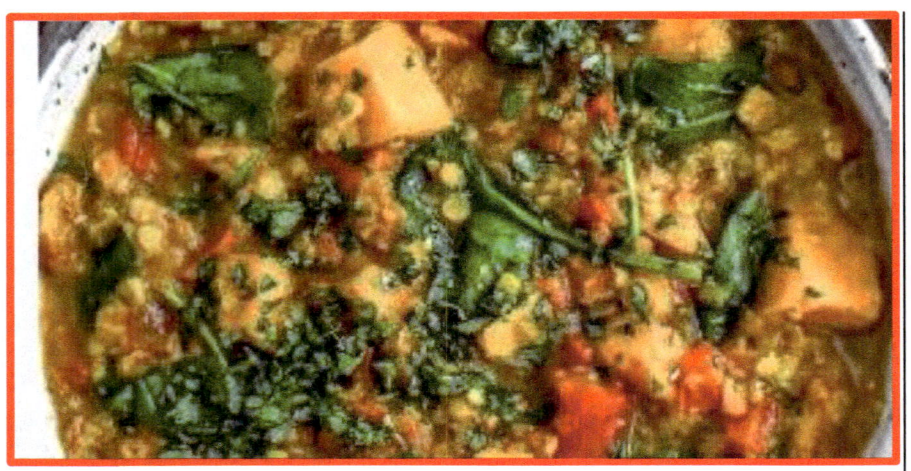

Time of Prep: 20 minutes
Cook Time: 30 minutes
Serving Size: 4 servings

Nutritional Information (per serving):
- Calories: 350
- Protein: 15g
- Fat: 12g
- Carbohydrates: 45g

Ingredients:

- 1 cup dried brown lentils, rinsed
- 2 cups low-sodium vegetable broth
- 1 medium sweet potato, peeled and cubed
- 1 tbsp olive oil
- 1 onion, diced
- 3 garlic cloves, minced
- 1 tbsp grated fresh ginger
- 2 tsp curry powder
- 1 tsp ground cumin
- 1/4 tsp cayenne pepper (optional)
- 1 cup canned diced tomatoes
- 1 cup unsweetened coconut milk
- Salt and pepper to taste
- Chopped cilantro for garnish (optional)

Instructions:

1. In a medium saucepan, combine the rinsed lentils and low-sodium vegetable broth. Bring the mixture to a boil, then reduce the heat to low, cover, and simmer for 15-20 minutes, or until the lentils are tender.

2. Meanwhile, in a large skillet, heat the olive oil over medium heat. Add the diced onion and sauté for 3-4 minutes, until translucent.

3. Add the minced garlic and grated ginger to the skillet and sauté for an additional minute, until fragrant.

4. Stir in the curry powder, ground cumin, and cayenne pepper (if using). Cook for 1 minute to toast the spices.

5. Add the cubed sweet potato, canned diced tomatoes, and unsweetened coconut milk to the skillet. Bring the mixture to a simmer and cook for 10-15 minutes, or until the sweet potato is tender.

6. Drain the cooked lentils and add them to the skillet. Stir to combine and let the curry simmer for an additional 5 minutes to allow the flavors to meld.

7. Season with salt and pepper to taste.

8. Serve the lentil and sweet potato curry over cooked brown rice or quinoa, garnished with chopped cilantro (if desired).

Lean Beef and Barley Soup

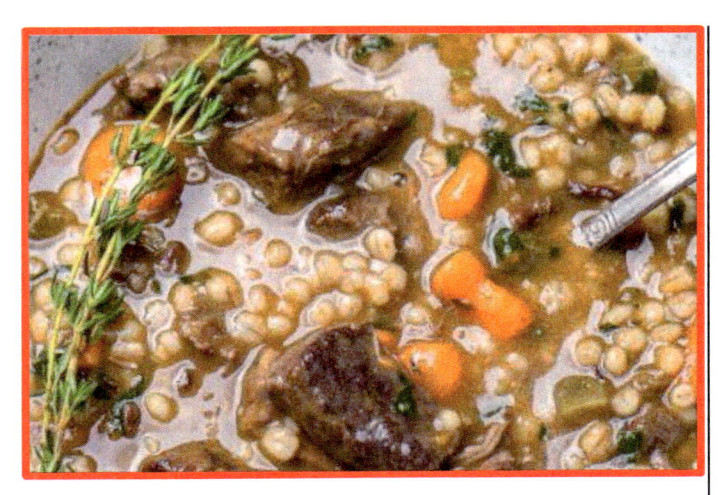

Time of Prep: 20 minutes
Cook Time: 45 minutes
Serving Size: 4 servings

Nutritional Information (per serving):
- Calories: 350
- Protein: 30g
- Fat: 10g
- Carbohydrates: 35g

Ingredients:

- 1 lb lean beef stew meat, cubed
- 1 tbsp olive oil
- 1 onion, diced
- 2 carrots, peeled and diced
- 2 celery stalks, diced
- 3 garlic cloves, minced
- 6 cups low-sodium beef broth
- 1 cup pearl barley
- 1 tsp dried thyme
- 1 cup sliced mushrooms

- 1 cup chopped green beans
- Salt and pepper to taste

Instructions:

1. In a large pot or Dutch oven, heat the olive oil over medium-high heat.
2. Add the cubed lean beef and brown it on all sides, about 5-7 minutes. Remove the beef from the pot and set it aside.
3. Reduce the heat to medium and add the diced onion, carrots, and celery to the pot. Sauté the vegetables for 5-7 minutes, or until they start to soften.
4. Add the minced garlic and sauté for an additional minute, until fragrant.
5. Pour in the low-sodium beef broth and stir in the pearl barley.
6. Return the browned beef to the pot and add the dried thyme.
7. Bring the soup to a boil, then reduce the heat to low, cover, and simmer for 30-40 minutes, or until the barley is tender and the beef is cooked through.
8. Stir in the sliced mushrooms and chopped green beans, and cook for an additional 5 minutes.
9. Season with salt and pepper to taste.
10. Serve hot.

Stuffed Bell Peppers with Turkey and Quinoa

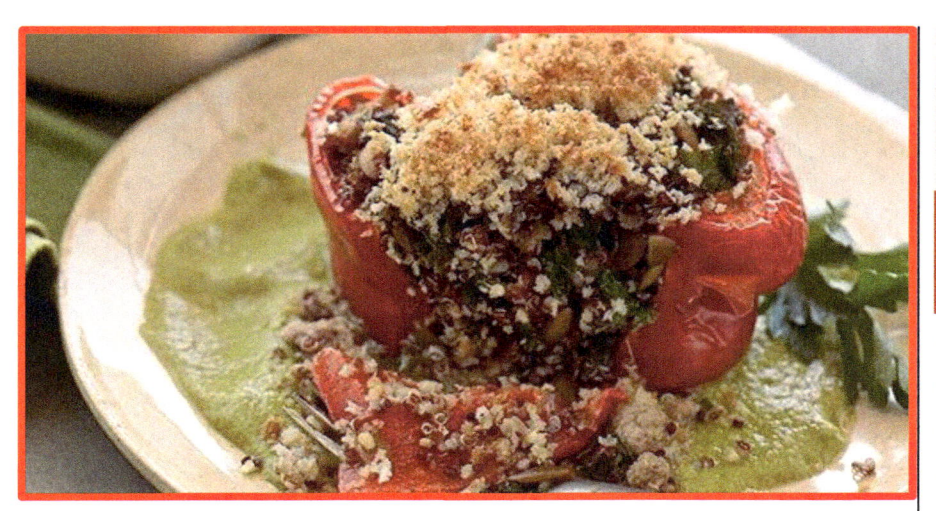

Time of Prep: 20 minutes
Cook Time: 40 minutes
Serving Size: 4 servings

Nutritional Information (per serving):
- Calories: 300
- Protein: 25g
- Fat: 10g
- Carbohydrates: 25g

Ingredients:

- 4 medium bell peppers, halved and seeded
- 1/2 lb lean ground turkey
- 1/2 lb lean ground chicken
- 1 cup cooked quinoa
- 1/2 cup diced onion
- 2 garlic cloves, minced
- 1 tsp dried oregano
- 1/4 tsp cayenne pepper (optional)
- 1 cup low-sodium tomato sauce
- 1/2 cup shredded low-fat mozzarella cheese

Instructions:

1. Preheat your oven to 375°F (190°C).
2. Arrange the bell pepper halves in a baking dish or on a rimmed baking sheet.
3. In a large bowl, combine the lean ground turkey, lean ground chicken, cooked quinoa, diced onion, minced garlic, dried oregano, and cayenne pepper (if using). Mix well.
4. Spoon the turkey-quinoa mixture evenly into the bell pepper halves.
5. Pour the low-sodium tomato sauce over the stuffed peppers.
6. Cover the baking dish with foil and bake for 30 minutes.

7. Remove the foil, sprinkle the shredded low-fat mozzarella cheese over the top, and bake for an additional 10 minutes, or until the peppers are tender and the cheese is melted.
8. Serve hot.

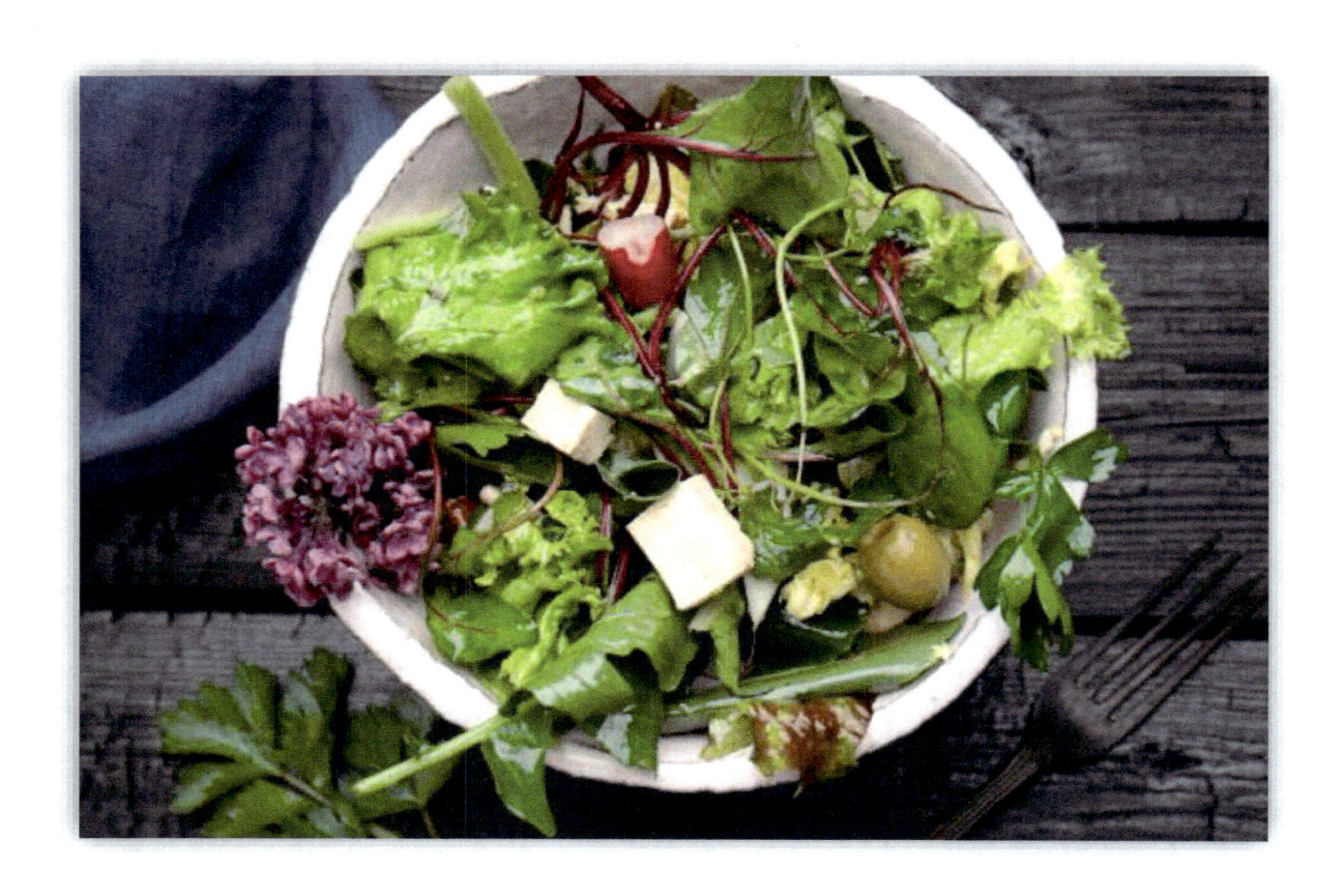

Tuna Salad Lettuce Wraps with Crunchy Vegetables

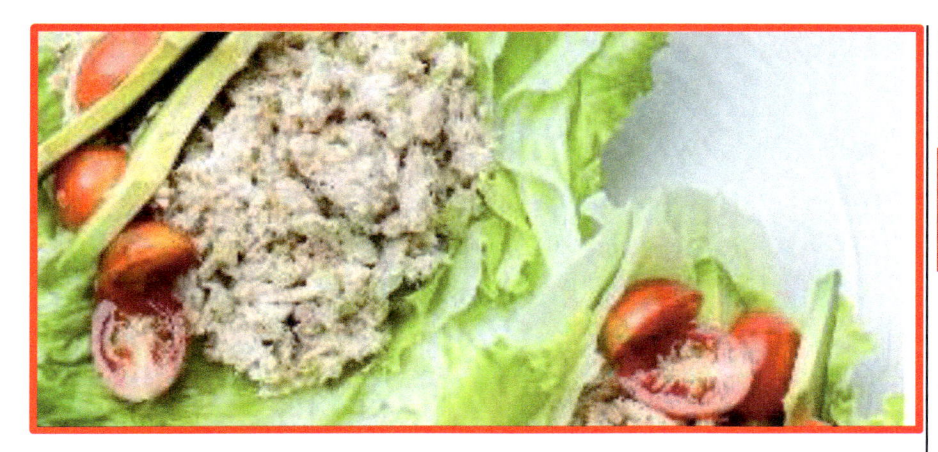

Time of Prep: 10 minutes
Cook Time: None
Serving Size: 2 servings

Nutritional Information (per serving):
- Calories: 150
- Protein: 20g
- Fat: 5g
- Carbohydrates: 5g

Ingredients:

- 1 (5 oz) can of water-packed tuna, drained
- 2 tbsp plain Greek yogurt
- 1 tbsp Dijon mustard
- 1 tbsp chopped celery
- 1 tbsp chopped red onion
- 1 tbsp diced cucumber
- 1 tsp lemon juice
- Salt and pepper to taste
- 4 large lettuce leaves (such as romaine or bibb)

Instructions:

1. In a medium bowl, combine the drained tuna, Greek yogurt, Dijon mustard, chopped celery, chopped red onion, diced cucumber, and lemon juice. Mix well.
2. Season the tuna salad with salt and pepper to taste.
3. Lay the large lettuce leaves on a flat surface.
4. Scoop the tuna salad evenly onto the center of each lettuce leaf.
5. Fold the sides of the lettuce leaf over the tuna salad and enjoy.

Baked Cod with Almond-Herb Topping

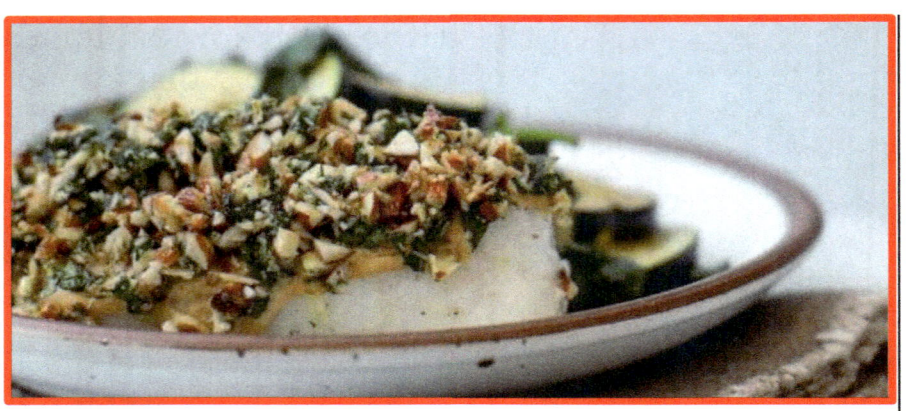

Time of Prep: 15 minutes
Cook Time: 20 minutes
Serving Size: 2 servings

Nutritional Information (per serving):
- Calories: 250
- Protein: 30g
- Fat: 10g
- Carbohydrates: 10g

Ingredients:

- 2 (4 oz) cod fillets
- 2 tbsp panko breadcrumbs
- 2 tbsp grated Parmesan cheese
- 2 tbsp chopped fresh parsley
- 2 tbsp chopped fresh dill
- 1 tbsp sliced almonds
- 1 tbsp olive oil
- 1 tbsp lemon juice
- Salt and pepper to taste

Instructions:

1. Preheat your oven to 400°F (200°C).
2. Place the cod fillets on a baking sheet lined with parchment paper.
3. In a small bowl, combine the panko breadcrumbs, grated Parmesan cheese, chopped parsley, chopped dill, and sliced almonds. Mix well.
4. Drizzle the olive oil and lemon juice over the cod fillets, then sprinkle the breadcrumb-almond mixture evenly over the top.
5. Bake the cod in the preheated oven for 18-20 minutes, or until the fish flakes easily with a fork and the topping is golden brown.
6. Serve the baked cod immediately, with a side of roasted sweet potato wedges or a fresh salad.

Vegetable Frittata with Feta and Spinach

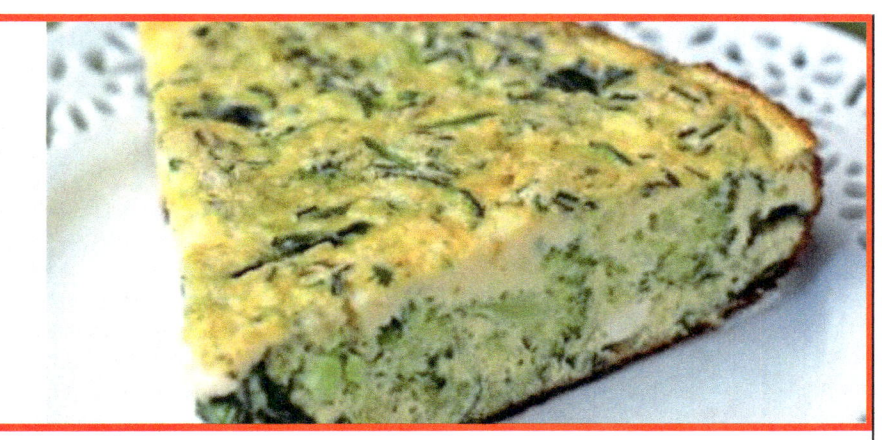

Time of Prep: 15 minutes
Cook Time: 20 minutes
Serving Size: 4 servings

Nutritional Information (per serving):

- Calories: 150
- Protein: 12g
- Fat: 8g
- Carbohydrates: 6g

Ingredients:

- 6 eggs
- 1/4 cup unsweetened almond milk
- 1 cup chopped spinach
- 1/2 cup diced bell pepper
- 1/2 cup diced onion
- 1/2 cup sliced mushrooms
- 1/2 cup diced tomatoes
- 2 tbsp crumbled feta cheese
- Salt and pepper to taste
- Cooking spray

Instructions:

1. Preheat your oven to 375°F (190°C).
2. In a medium bowl, whisk the eggs and almond milk together. Season with a pinch of salt and pepper.
3. Coat a 9-inch oven-safe non-stick skillet with cooking spray and place it over medium heat.
4. Add the chopped spinach, diced bell pepper, diced onion, sliced mushrooms, and diced tomatoes to the skillet. Sauté the vegetables for 3-4 minutes, until they start to soften.
5. Pour the whisked egg mixture over the vegetables in the skillet, making sure to evenly distribute the vegetables.
6. Sprinkle the crumbled feta cheese over the top of the frittata.
7. Transfer the skillet to the preheated oven and bake for 15-20 minutes, or until the frittata is set and the cheese is melted.

8. Remove the frittata from the oven and let it cool for a few minutes before slicing and serving.

Turkey Meatballs with Whole Wheat Pasta and Steamed Broccoli

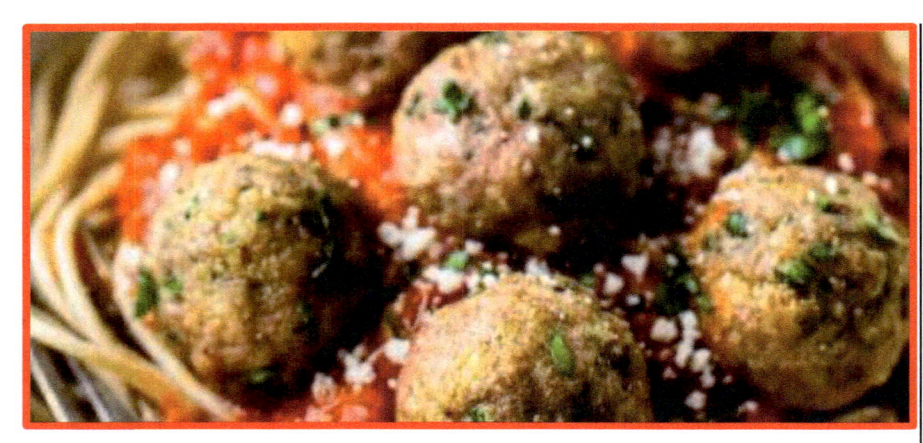

Time of Prep: 20 minutes
Cook Time: 30 minutes
Serving Size: 4 servings

Nutritional Information (per serving):
- Calories: 400
- Protein: 30g
- Fat: 12g
- Carbohydrates: 40g

Ingredients:

- 1/2 lb lean ground turkey
- 1/2 lb lean ground chicken
- 1/2 cup whole wheat breadcrumbs
- 1 egg, lightly beaten
- 2 tbsp grated Parmesan cheese
- 2 garlic cloves, minced
- 1 tsp dried oregano
- 1/4 tsp red pepper flakes (optional)
- Salt and pepper to taste
- 8 oz whole wheat pasta
- 1 cup low-sodium marinara sauce
- 2 cups broccoli florets, steamed

Instructions:

1. Preheat your oven to 400°F (200°C).
2. In a large bowl, combine the lean ground turkey, lean ground chicken, whole wheat breadcrumbs, beaten egg, grated Parmesan cheese, minced garlic, dried oregano, and red pepper flakes (if using). Mix well and season with salt and pepper.
3. Roll the turkey-chicken mixture into 1-inch meatballs and place them on a baking sheet lined with parchment paper.

57 | Gout Diet for Seniors

4. Bake the meatballs in the preheated oven for 20-25 minutes, or until they are cooked through and lightly browned.
5. While the meatballs are baking, cook the whole wheat pasta according to the package instructions. Drain and set aside.
6. In a saucepan, heat the low-sodium marinara sauce over medium heat until warmed through.
7. Add the cooked meatballs to the marinara sauce and stir to coat.
8. Serve the turkey meatballs and sauce over the cooked whole wheat pasta, accompanied by the steamed broccoli florets.

Creamy Butternut Squash Soup with Toasted Pumpkin Seeds

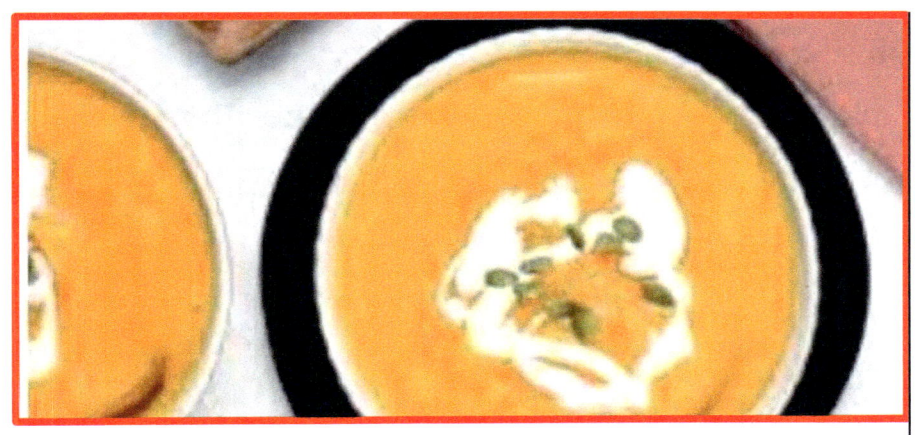

Time of Prep: 20 minutes
Cook Time: 45 minutes
Serving Size: 4 servings

Nutritional Information (per serving):
- Calories: 150
- Protein: 4g
- Fat: 5g
- Carbohydrates: 22g

Ingredients:

- 1 medium butternut squash, peeled, seeded, and cubed (about 4 cups)
- 1 tbsp olive oil
- 1 onion, diced
- 2 garlic cloves, minced
- 4 cups low-sodium vegetable broth
- 1 cup unsweetened almond milk

- 1 tsp ground cinnamon
- 1/4 tsp ground nutmeg
- 1/4 tsp ground ginger
- Salt and pepper to taste
- 2 tbsp toasted pumpkin seeds for garnish
- Chopped fresh parsley for garnish (optional)

Instructions:

1. In a large pot or Dutch oven, heat the olive oil over medium heat.
2. Add the diced onion and sauté for 3-4 minutes, until translucent.
3. Add the minced garlic and sauté for an additional minute, until fragrant.
4. Add the cubed butternut squash and low-sodium vegetable broth to the pot. Bring the mixture to a boil, then reduce the heat to low, cover, and simmer for 30-35 minutes, or until the squash is very soft.
5. Remove the pot from heat and use an immersion blender to puree the soup until smooth. Alternatively, you can transfer the soup to a blender in batches and blend until smooth.
6. Stir in the unsweetened almond milk, ground cinnamon, ground nutmeg, and ground ginger. Season with salt and pepper to taste.
7. Reheat the soup over medium heat, if necessary, until warmed through.
8. Serve the butternut squash soup hot, garnished with toasted pumpkin seeds and chopped fresh parsley (if desired).

Chapter 7: Side Dish and Snack Recipes (Healthy and enjoyable options)

In this collection of gout-friendly side dishes and snacks tailored for seniors, we have curated a selection of nutritious and delicious recipes designed to support gout management while delighting the taste buds. Each recipe has been thoughtfully crafted to incorporate ingredients that are low in purines, a key factor in managing gout, and high in essential nutrients to promote overall health and well-being.

These recipes offer a variety of flavors and textures, from spiced roasted chickpeas to mango salsa with whole grain pita chips, providing seniors with satisfying options that are gentle on their joints. By focusing on simple and accessible ingredients, these dishes aim to make healthy eating enjoyable and sustainable for individuals managing gout.

Nutritionally, these recipes are rich in protein, fiber, vitamins, and minerals, essential for supporting joint health and reducing inflammation associated with gout. By incorporating a variety of fruits, vegetables, whole grains, and lean proteins, these dishes offer a well-rounded approach to gout management, helping seniors maintain a balanced and nutritious diet.

Whether enjoyed as a side dish, snack, or light meal, these gout-friendly recipes aim to empower seniors to make informed and delicious choices that support their overall health and well-being. With a focus on flavor, variety, and nutrient density, these dishes offer a holistic approach to gout management, ensuring that seniors can savor their meals while taking care of their bodies.

Spiced Roasted Chickpeas

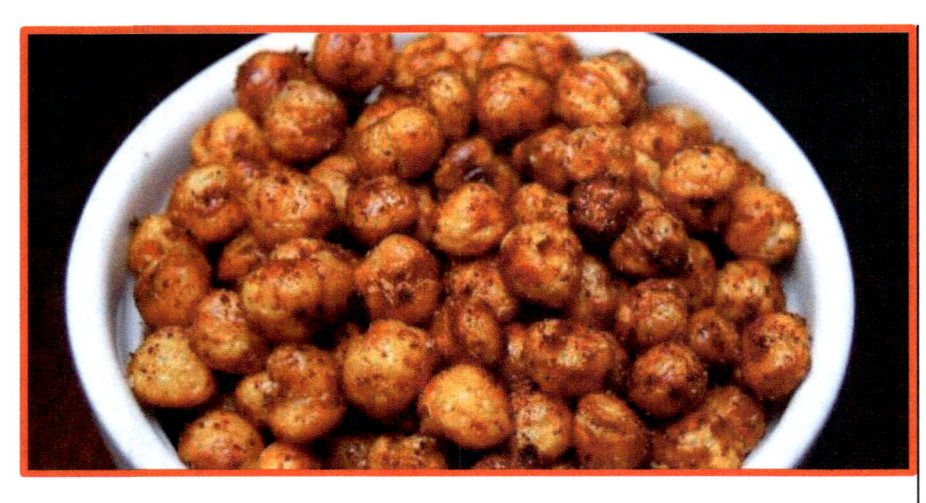

Time of Prep: 10 minutes
Cook Time: 25 minutes
Serving Size: 4 servings

Nutritional Information (per serving):
- Calories: 120
- Protein: 6g
- Fat: 5g
- Carbohydrates: 15g

Ingredients:

- 1 (15 oz) can of low-sodium chickpeas, drained and rinsed
- 1 tbsp olive oil
- 1 tsp paprika
- 1/2 tsp garlic powder
- 1/4 tsp cayenne pepper (optional)
- 1/4 tsp ground cumin
- Salt and pepper to taste

Instructions:

1. Preheat your oven to 400°F (200°C).
2. Pat the drained and rinsed chickpeas dry with a paper towel.
3. In a bowl, toss the chickpeas with the olive oil, paprika, garlic powder, cayenne pepper (if using), and ground cumin. Season with a pinch of salt and pepper.
4. Spread the seasoned chickpeas in a single layer on a baking sheet.
5. Roast the chickpeas in the preheated oven for 20-25 minutes, stirring halfway, until they are crispy and golden brown.
6. Remove the roasted chickpeas from the oven and let them cool for a few minutes before serving.

Caprese Skewers with Balsamic Drizzle

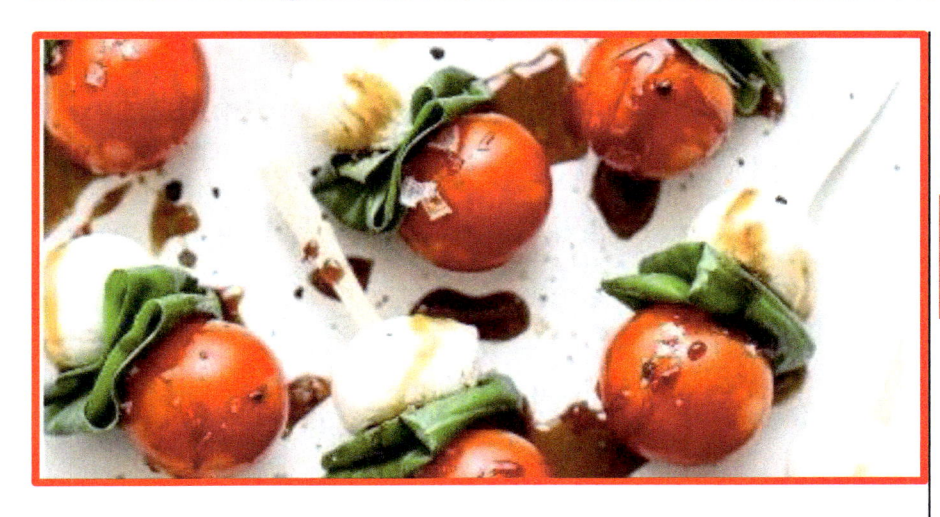

Time of Prep: 15 minutes
Cook Time: None
Serving Size: 4 servings

Nutritional Information (per serving):
- Calories: 100
- Protein: 6g
- Fat: 6g
- Carbohydrates: 6g

Ingredients:

- 12 cherry tomatoes
- 12 small fresh mozzarella balls
- 12 fresh basil leaves
- 1 tbsp high-quality balsamic vinegar
- Salt and pepper to taste

Instructions:

1. Thread the cherry tomatoes, mozzarella balls, and fresh basil leaves onto small skewers, alternating the ingredients.
2. Arrange the Caprese skewers on a serving platter.
3. Drizzle the balsamic vinegar over the skewers.
4. Season with a pinch of salt and pepper.
5. Serve immediately or chill in the refrigerator until ready to serve.

Greek Yogurt Dip with Crunchy Veggies

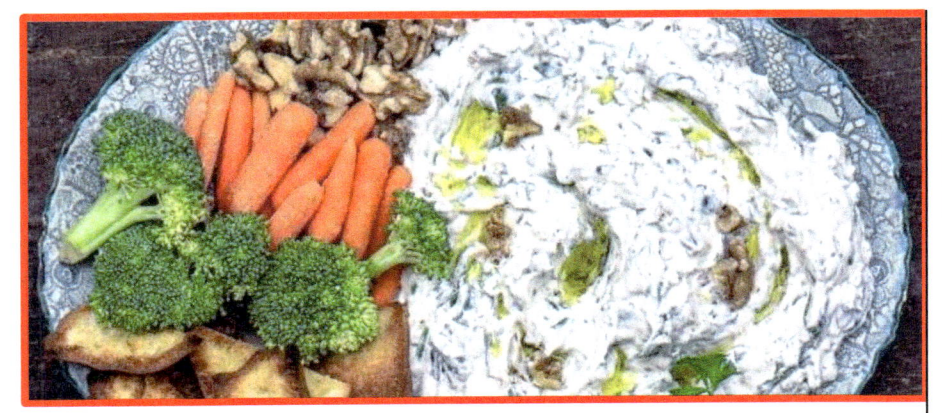

Time of Prep: 10 mins
Cook Time: None
Serving Size: 4 servings

Nutritional Information:
- Calories: 80
- Protein: 8g
- Fat: 3g
- Carbohydrates: 5g

Gout Diet for Seniors

Ingredients:

- 1 cup plain Greek yogurt
- 2 tbsp chopped fresh dill
- 1 tbsp lemon juice
- 1 garlic clove, minced
- 1/4 tsp salt
- Assorted raw vegetables (such as carrot sticks, cucumber slices, and bell pepper strips)

Instructions:

1. In a small bowl, combine the plain Greek yogurt, chopped fresh dill, lemon juice, minced garlic, and salt. Stir well to mix.
2. Serve the Greek yogurt dip with a variety of raw vegetables, such as carrot sticks, cucumber slices, and bell pepper strips.
3. Refrigerate any leftover dip in an airtight container for up to 3 days.

Quinoa and Feta Stuffed Bell Peppers

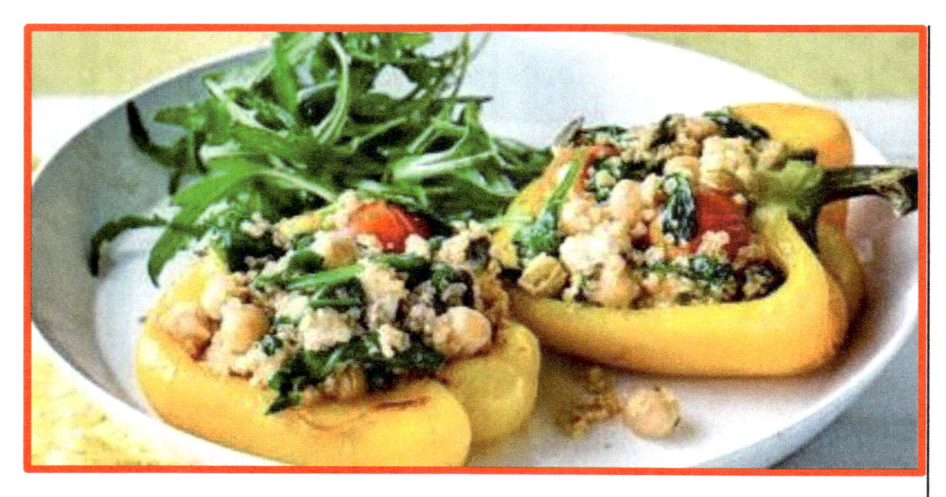

Time of Prep: 20 minutes
Cook Time: 30 minutes
Serving Size: 4 servings

Nutritional Information (per serving):

- Calories: 150
- Protein: 7g
- Fat: 7g
- Carbohydrates: 18g

Ingredients:

- 4 medium bell peppers, halved and seeded
- 1/2 cup cooked quinoa
- 1/2 cup cooked brown rice
- 1/2 cup diced tomatoes
- 2 tbsp crumbled low-fat feta cheese
- 2 tbsp chopped fresh parsley
- 1 tbsp olive oil
- Salt and pepper to taste

Instructions:

1. Preheat your oven to 375°F (190°C).
2. Arrange the bell pepper halves in a baking dish or on a rimmed baking sheet.
3. In a medium bowl, combine the cooked quinoa, cooked brown rice, diced tomatoes, crumbled low-fat feta cheese, and chopped fresh parsley. Mix well.
4. Spoon the quinoa-rice mixture evenly into the bell pepper halves.
5. Drizzle the olive oil over the stuffed peppers and season with salt and pepper.
6. Bake the stuffed peppers in the preheated oven for 25-30 minutes, or until the peppers are tender and the filling is heated through.
7. Serve the quinoa and feta stuffed bell peppers warm.

Fruit Salad with Honey-Lime Dressing

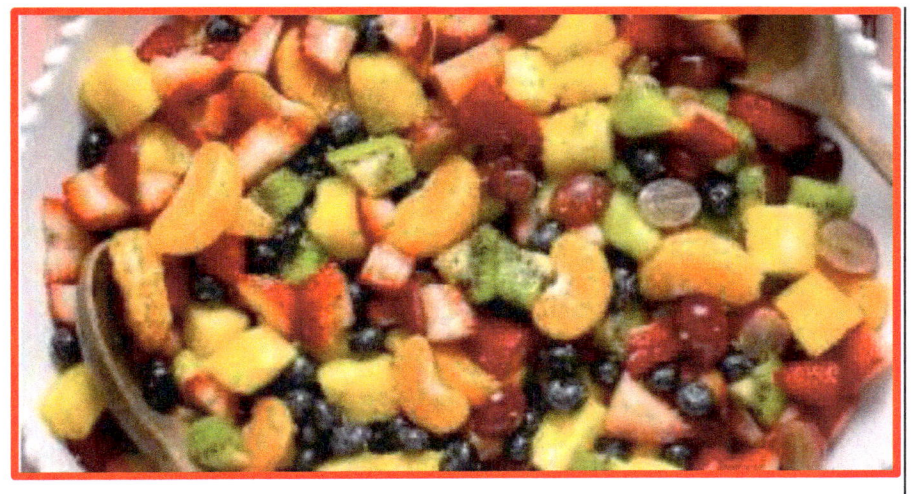

Time of Prep: 15 minutes
Cook Time: None
Serving Size: 4 servings

Nutritional Information (per serving):
- Calories: 80
- Protein: 1g
- Fat: 0g
- Carbohydrates: 20g

Ingredients:

- 2 cups mixed fresh fruit (such as pineapple, mango, strawberries, and blueberries)
- 1 tbsp maple syrup
- 1 tbsp lime juice
- 1 tsp lime zest
- Pinch of salt

Instructions:

1. In a large bowl, combine the mixed fresh fruit.
2. In a small bowl, whisk together the maple syrup, lime juice, lime zest, and a pinch of salt.
3. Drizzle the honey-lime dressing over the fruit salad and gently toss to coat.
4. Serve the fruit salad immediately or chill in the refrigerator until ready to serve.

Cucumber Avocado Rolls with Herbs

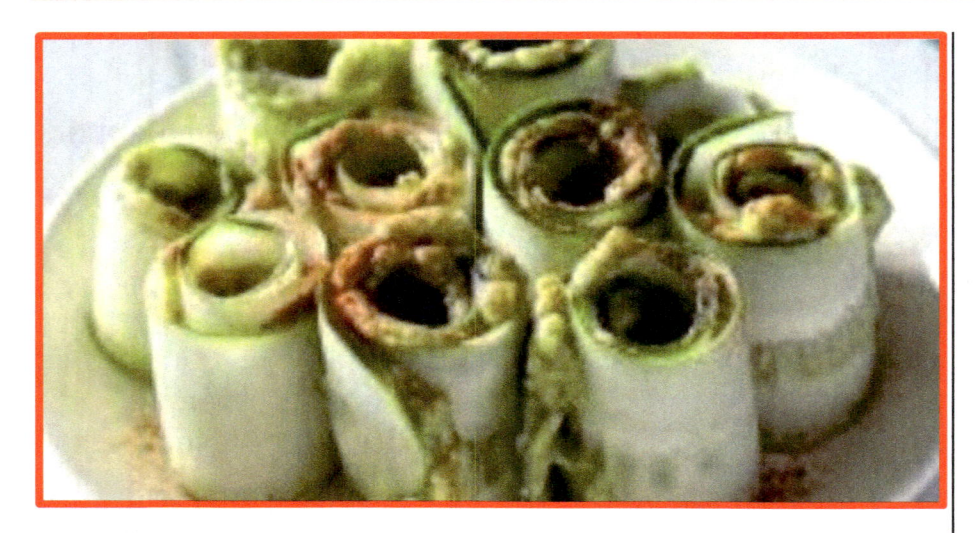

Time of Prep: 20 minutes
Cook Time: None
Serving Size: 4 servings

Nutritional Information (per serving):
- Calories: 70
- Protein: 1g
- Fat: 5g
- Carbohydrates: 6g

Ingredients:

- 1 large cucumber, peeled and sliced lengthwise into thin strips
- 1 ripe avocado, sliced
- 2 tbsp chopped fresh cilantro
- 1 tbsp chopped fresh dill
- 1 tbsp lime juice
- Salt and pepper to taste

Instructions:

1. Lay the cucumber strips on a flat surface, with the skin side facing down.
2. Place a few slices of avocado near the bottom of each cucumber strip.

3. Sprinkle the chopped fresh cilantro and dill over the avocado.
4. Drizzle the lime juice over the avocado and herbs.
5. Season with a pinch of salt and pepper.
6. Carefully roll up the cucumber strips, starting from the bottom and rolling towards the top.
7. Secure the rolls with toothpicks, if needed.
8. Serve the cucumber avocado rolls immediately or chill in the refrigerator until ready to serve.

Crispy Baked Sweet Potato Fries

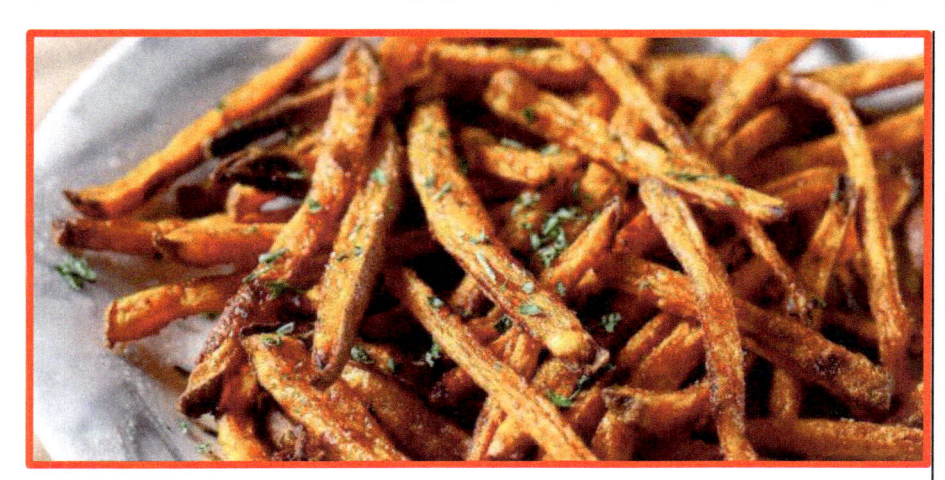

Time of Prep: 15 minutes
Cook Time: 25 minutes
Serving Size: 4 servings

Nutritional Information (per serving):
- Calories: 100
- Protein: 2g
- Fat: 4g
- Carbohydrates: 15g

Ingredients:

- 2 medium sweet potatoes, peeled and cut into 1/2-inch thick fries
- 1 tbsp olive oil
- 1 tsp paprika
- 1/2 tsp garlic powder
- 1/4 tsp ground cumin
- Salt and pepper to taste

Instructions:

1. Preheat your oven to 400°F (200°C).
2. In a large bowl, toss the sweet potato fries with the olive oil, paprika, garlic powder, and ground cumin. Season with a pinch of salt and pepper.
3. Spread the seasoned sweet potato fries in a single layer on a baking sheet lined with parchment paper.

4. Bake the fries in the preheated oven for 20-25 minutes, flipping them halfway, until they are crispy and golden brown.
5. Remove the baked sweet potato fries from the oven and let them cool for a few minutes before serving.

Edamame with Lemon Pepper Seasoning

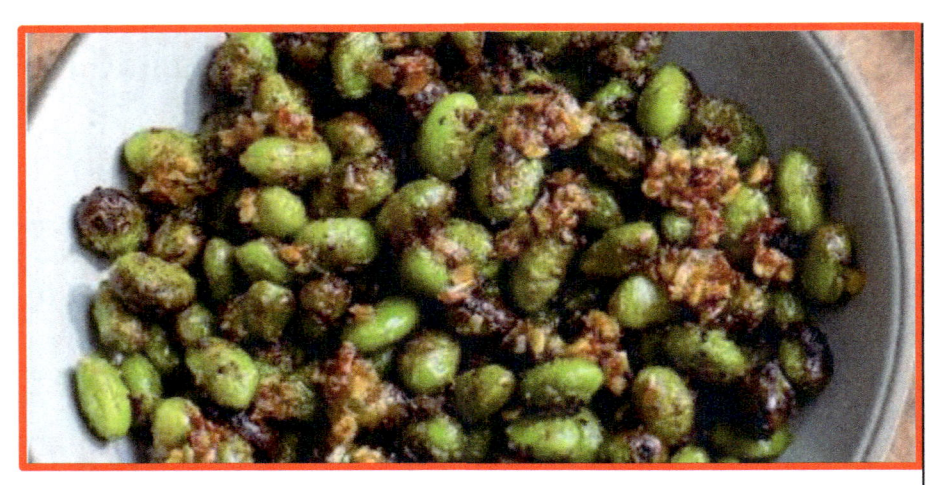

Time of Prep: 5 minutes
Cook Time: 5 minutes
Serving Size: 2 servings

Nutritional Information (per serving):
- Calories: 100
- Protein: 10g
- Fat: 5g
- Carbohydrates: 8g

Ingredients:

- 1 cup frozen edamame, in the pod
- 1 tsp lemon pepper seasoning

Instructions:

1. Bring a small pot of water to a boil.
2. Add the frozen edamame to the boiling water and cook for 4-5 minutes, or until the edamame is tender.
3. Drain the cooked edamame and transfer it to a serving bowl.
4. Sprinkle the lemon pepper seasoning over the edamame and toss gently to coat.
5. Serve the edamame warm, with the pods intact, allowing the eaters to pop the beans out of the pods.

Mango Salsa with Whole Grain Pita Chips

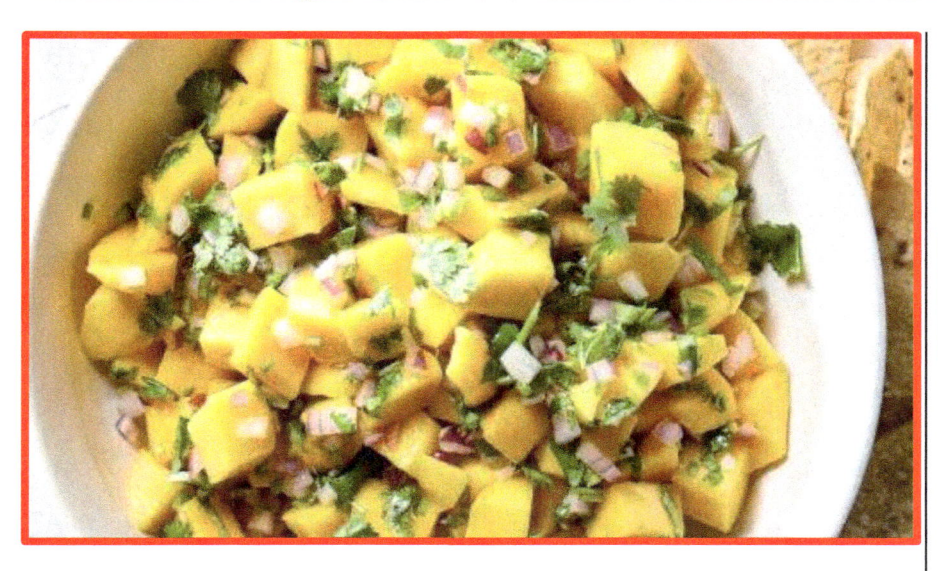

Time of Prep: 20 minutes
Cook Time: 10 minutes
Serving Size: 4 servings

Nutritional Information (per serving):

- Calories: 150
- Protein: 4g
- Fat: 5g
- Carbohydrates: 22g

Ingredients:

- 1 ripe mango, diced
- 1/2 red onion, finely chopped
- 1 jalapeño, seeded and finely chopped (optional)
- 2 tbsp chopped fresh cilantro
- 1 tbsp lime juice
- 1/4 tsp salt
- 4 whole grain pita breads, cut into wedges
- 1 tbsp olive oil

Instructions:

1. Preheat your oven to 400°F (200°C).
2. In a medium bowl, combine the diced mango, chopped red onion, chopped jalapeño (if using), chopped fresh cilantro, lime juice, and salt. Stir to mix well.
3. Arrange the whole grain pita wedges on a baking sheet. Brush the pita wedges lightly with olive oil.
4. Bake the pita wedges in the preheated oven for 8-10 minutes, or until they are crispy and lightly golden.
5. Remove the baked pita chips from the oven and let them cool for a few minutes.
6. Serve the mango salsa with the baked whole grain pita chips.

Spinach and Feta Stuffed Mushrooms

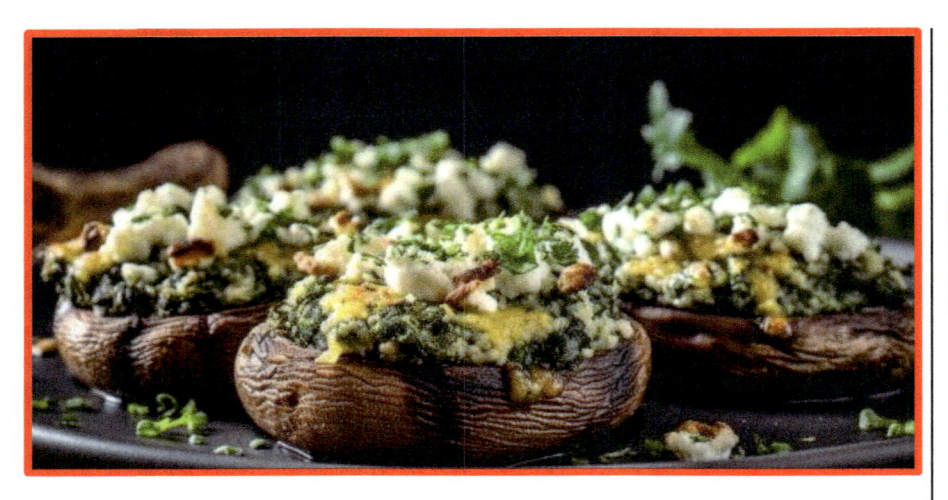

Time of Prep: 15 minutes
Cook Time: 20 minutes
Serving Size: 4 servings

Nutritional Information (per serving):
- Calories: 80
- Protein: 5g
- Fat: 5g
- Carbohydrates: 4g

Ingredients:

- 12 medium-sized mushrooms, stems removed and chopped
- 1 cup fresh spinach, chopped
- 1 oz crumbled low-fat feta cheese
- 1 oz shredded low-fat mozzarella cheese
- 1 tbsp olive oil
- 1 garlic clove, minced
- Salt and pepper to taste

Instructions:

1. Preheat the oven to 375°F (190°C).
2. In a skillet, heat the olive oil over medium heat. Add the chopped mushroom stems and minced garlic. Sauté for 2-3 minutes until fragrant.
3. Add the chopped spinach to the skillet and sauté until wilted, about 2 minutes.
4. Remove the skillet from heat and stir in the crumbled low-fat feta cheese and shredded low-fat mozzarella cheese. Season with salt and pepper.
5. Stuff the mushroom caps with the spinach-cheese mixture.
6. Place the stuffed mushrooms on a baking sheet and bake for 15-20 minutes, or until the mushrooms are tender and the filling is heated through.
7. Serve the spinach and feta stuffed mushrooms warm.

Chapter 8: Dessert Recipes (Sweet treats without compromising gout management)

Who says you have to give up desserts to manage gout? This chapter is dedicated to satisfying your sweet tooth with delicious treats that won't compromise your health. These recipes are crafted with low-purine ingredients and smart swaps to help you enjoy dessert without worrying about triggering a gout flare. From fruity delights to creamy indulgences and chocolatey goodness, you'll find a variety of options to satisfy your cravings while keeping your gout in check. So go ahead and indulge in a little sweetness – the smart way!

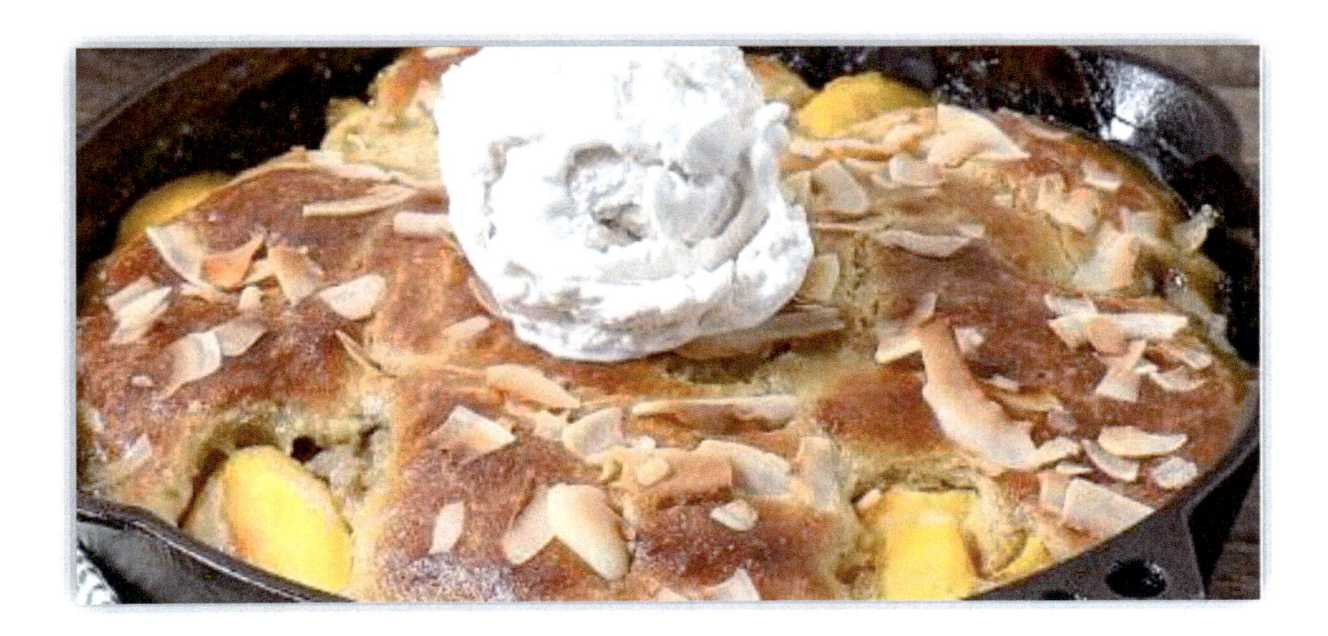

Easy Applesauce

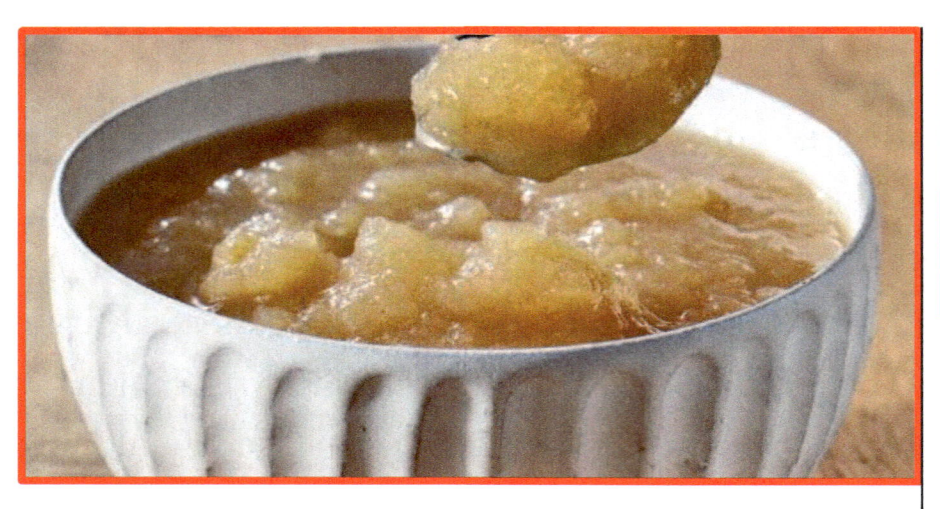

Time of Prep: 10 mins
Cook Time: 20 minutes
Serving Size: 4 servings

Nutritional Information (per serving):
- Calories: 80
- Carbohydrates: 20g

Ingredients:

- 4 medium apples, peeled, cored, and chopped
- 1/4 cup water
- 1 tsp ground cinnamon
- 1 tbsp honey (optional)

Instructions:

1. In a medium saucepan, combine the chopped apples and water.
2. Bring the mixture to a boil over medium heat, then reduce the heat to low, cover, and simmer for 15-20 minutes, or until the apples are very soft.
3. Remove the saucepan from heat and let the apples cool slightly.
4. Using a potato masher or an immersion blender, mash or puree the cooked apples until you reach your desired consistency.
5. Stir in the ground cinnamon and honey (if using) until well combined.
6. Serve the homemade applesauce warm or chilled.

Graham Cracker Delight

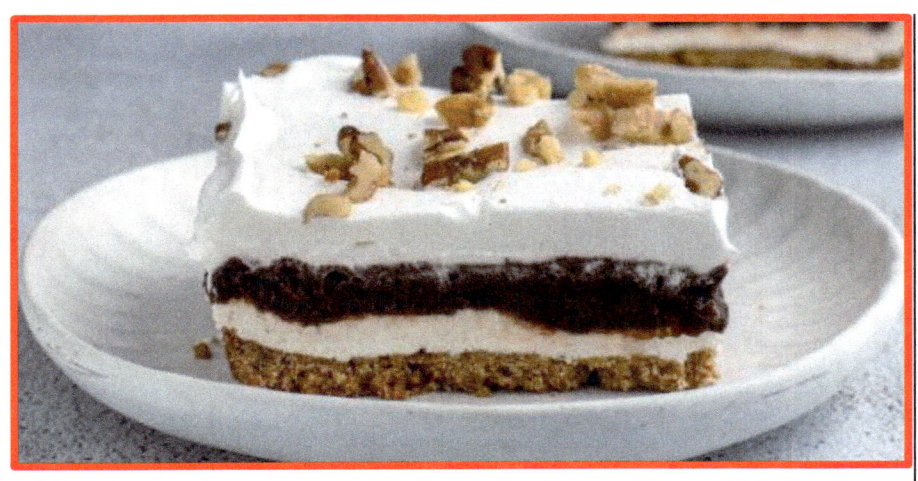

Time of Prep: 15 minutes
Cook Time: None
Serving Size: 4 servings

Nutritional Information (per serving):

- Calories: 200
- Protein: 8g
- Fat: 5g
- Carbohydrates: 30g

Ingredients:

- 8 whole graham crackers, broken into pieces
- 1 cup low-fat ricotta cheese
- 1/4 cup honey
- 1 tsp vanilla extract
- 1/2 cup fresh berries (such as blueberries or raspberries)

Instructions:

1. In a medium bowl, combine the broken graham cracker pieces, low-fat ricotta cheese, honey, and vanilla extract. Stir until well mixed.

2. Gently fold in the fresh berries, being careful not to crush them.

3. Serve the graham cracker delight immediately or chill in the refrigerator until ready to serve.

Lazy Apple Crisp

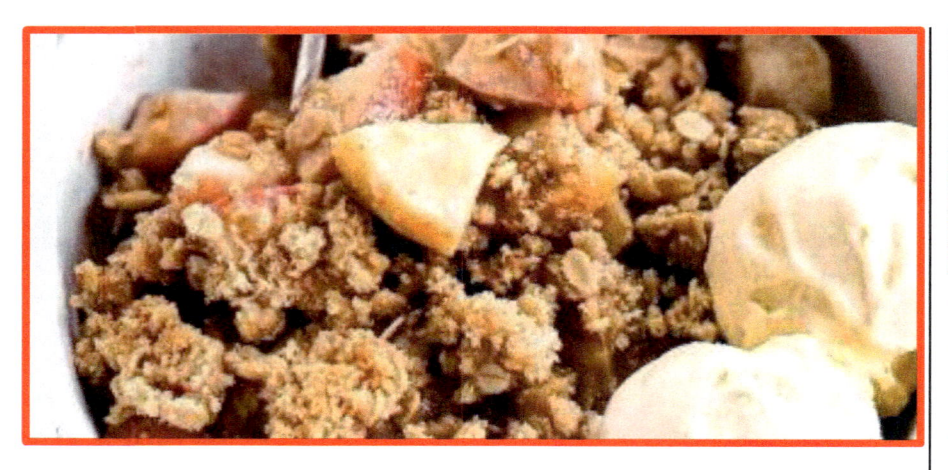

Time of Prep: 15 minutes
Cook Time: 30 minutes
Serving Size: 4 servings

Nutritional Information (per serving):
- Calories: 180
- Protein: 2g
- Fat: 6g
- Carbohydrates: 30g

Ingredients:

- 4 medium apples, peeled, cored, and sliced
- 1/2 cup rolled oats
- 2 tbsp whole wheat flour
- 2 tbsp brown sugar
- 1 tsp ground cinnamon
- 2 tbsp unsalted butter, melted

Instructions:

1. Preheat your oven to 375°F (190°C).
2. Arrange the sliced apples in a baking dish.
3. In a small bowl, combine the rolled oats, whole wheat flour, brown sugar, and ground cinnamon. Mix well.
4. Drizzle the melted unsalted butter over the oat mixture and stir until the ingredients are evenly coated.
5. Sprinkle the oat topping over the sliced apples in the baking dish.
6. Bake the lazy apple crisp in the preheated oven for 25-30 minutes, or until the apples are tender and the topping is golden brown.
7. Serve the lazy apple crisp warm, or let it cool slightly before serving.

Berry Cherry Smoothie

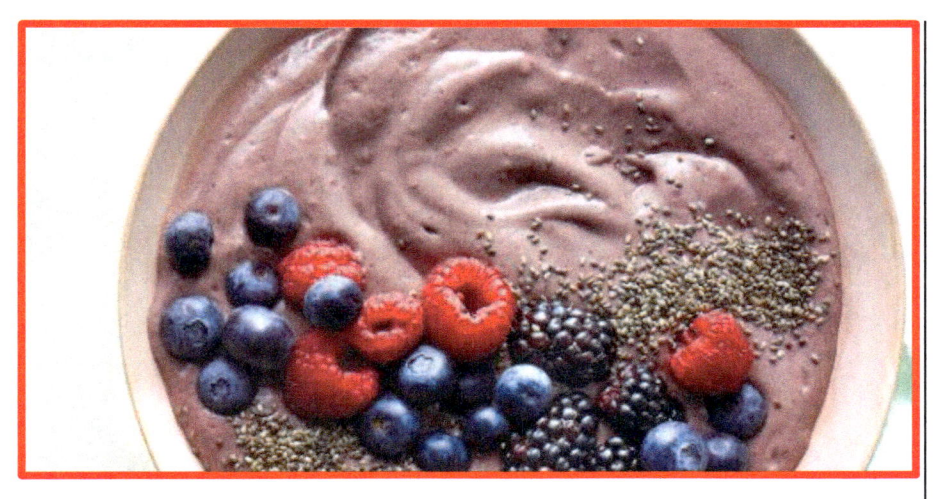

Time of Prep: 10 mins
Cook Time: None
Serving Size: 2 servings

Nutritional Information (per serving):
- Calories: 150
- Protein: 8g
- Fat: 2g
- Carbohydrates: 22g

Ingredients:

- 1 cup frozen mixed berries (such as blueberries, raspberries, and blackberries)
- 1/2 cup frozen cherries
- 1 cup unsweetened almond milk
- 1/2 cup plain Greek yogurt
- 1 tbsp honey (optional)

Instructions:

1. In a high-speed blender, combine the frozen mixed berries, frozen cherries, unsweetened almond milk, and plain Greek yogurt.
2. Blend the ingredients on high speed until the smoothie is smooth and creamy.
3. Taste the smoothie and add the honey (if using) to adjust the sweetness to your preference.
4. Pour the berry cherry smoothie into two glasses and serve immediately.

Gooey Blueberry Oat Bars

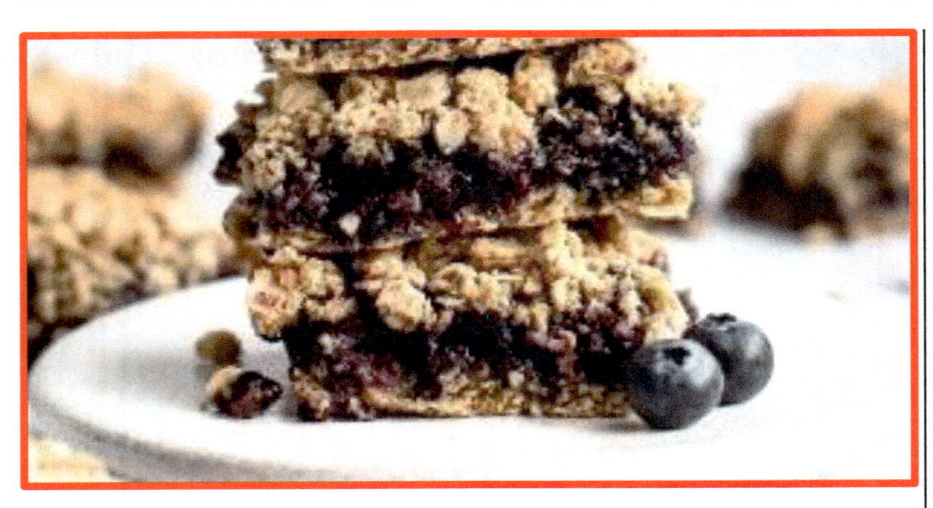

Time of Prep: 20 minutes
Cook Time: 30 minutes
Serving Size: 9 bars

Nutritional Information (per bar):
- Calories: 150
- Protein: 3g
- Fat: 6g
- Carbohydrates: 22g

Ingredients:

- 1 cup rolled oats
- 1/2 cup whole wheat flour
- 1/4 cup brown sugar
- 1/4 tsp ground cinnamon
- 1/4 tsp salt
- 4 tbsp unsalted butter, melted
- 1 cup fresh or frozen blueberries
- 2 tbsp honey

Instructions:

1. Preheat your oven to 350°F (175°C).
2. In a medium bowl, combine the rolled oats, whole wheat flour, brown sugar, ground cinnamon, and salt. Mix well.
3. Stir in the melted unsalted butter until the dry ingredients are evenly coated.
4. Press half of the oat mixture into an 8x8-inch baking dish, creating a bottom crust.
5. Spread the fresh or frozen blueberries evenly over the bottom crust.
6. Drizzle the honey over the blueberries.
7. Sprinkle the remaining oat mixture over the top of the blueberries, gently pressing it down.
8. Bake the gooey blueberry oat bars in the preheated oven for 25-30 minutes, or until the top is golden brown.
9. Allow the bars to cool completely before cutting and serving.

Chocolate Covered Strawberries

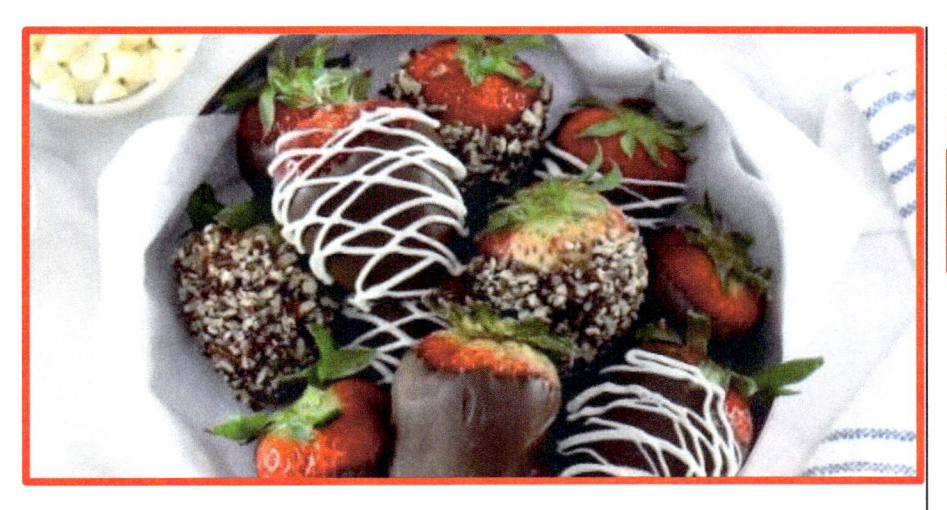

Time of Prep: 15 minutes
Cook Time: None
Serving Size: 8 servings

Nutritional Information (per serving):
- Calories: 60
- Protein: 1g
- Fat: 3g
- Carbohydrates: 8g

Ingredients:

- 16 fresh strawberries
- 2 oz dark chocolate, chopped
- 1 tsp coconut oil (optional)

Instructions:

1. Wash and thoroughly dry the fresh strawberries, leaving a small amount of the stem attached.
2. In a small microwave-safe bowl, combine the chopped dark chocolate and coconut oil (if using). Microwave in 30-second intervals, stirring between each interval, until the chocolate is melted and smooth.
3. Carefully dip each strawberry into the melted chocolate, coating about three-quarters of the berry.
4. Place the chocolate-dipped strawberries on a parchment-lined baking sheet or plate.
5. Refrigerate the chocolate-covered strawberries for at least 30 minutes, or until the chocolate has hardened.
6. Serve the chocolate-covered strawberries chilled.

Better-for-You Peanut Butter Brownies

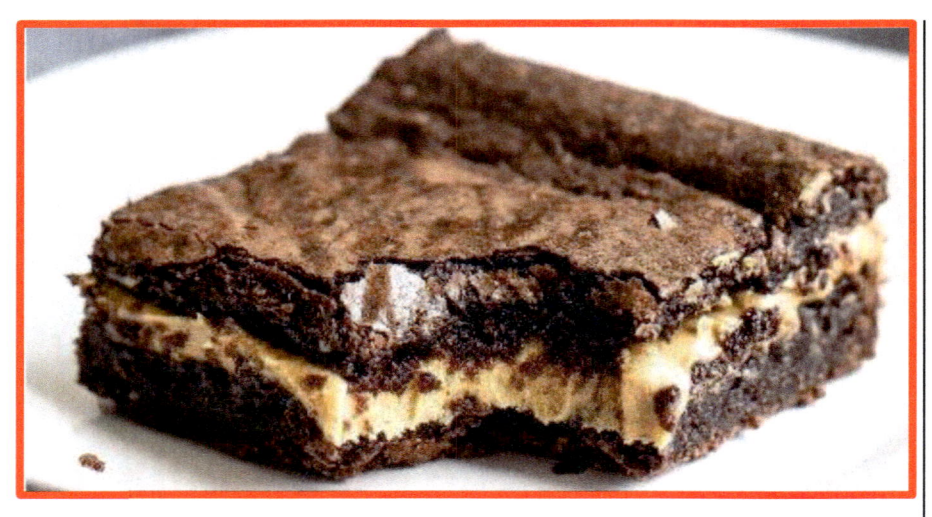

Time of Prep: 20 minutes
Cook Time: 25 minutes
Serving Size: 16 brownies

Nutritional Information (per brownie):

- Calories: 100
- Protein: 3g
- Fat: 5g
- Carbohydrates: 12g

Ingredients:

- 1/2 cup whole wheat flour
- 1/4 cup unsweetened cocoa powder
- 1/2 tsp baking powder
- 1/4 tsp salt
- 1/2 cup natural peanut butter
- 1/2 cup honey
- 2 eggs
- 1 tsp vanilla extract

Instructions:

1. Preheat your oven to 350°F (175°C).
2. Grease an 8x8-inch baking pan with non-stick cooking spray.
3. In a medium bowl, whisk together the whole wheat flour, unsweetened cocoa powder, baking powder, and salt.
4. In a separate bowl, combine the natural peanut butter, honey, eggs, and vanilla extract. Mix until well blended.
5. Gradually add the dry ingredients to the wet ingredients, stirring just until combined.
6. Spread the brownie batter evenly into the prepared baking pan.
7. Bake the brownies in the preheated oven for 22-25 minutes, or until a toothpick inserted into the center comes out clean.
8. Allow the brownies to cool completely before cutting into squares.

Creamy Avocado Pudding

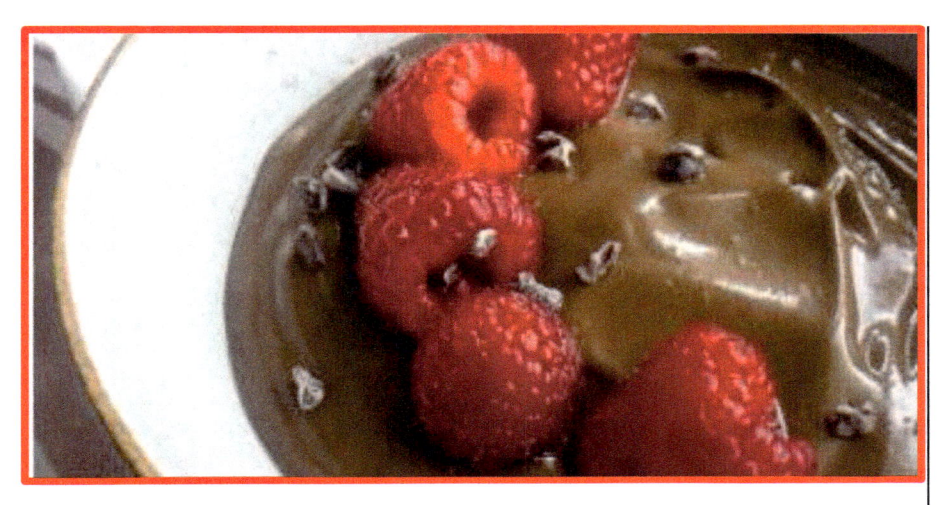

Time of Prep: 10 minutes
Cook Time: None
Serving Size: 4 servings

Nutritional Information (per serving):
- Calories: 120
- Protein: 2g
- Fat: 8g
- Carbohydrates: 12g

Ingredients:

- 1 ripe avocado, pitted and peeled
- 1/2 cup unsweetened almond milk
- 2 tbsp honey
- 1 tbsp unsweetened cocoa powder
- 1 tsp vanilla extract
- Pinch of salt

Instructions:

1. In a food processor or high-speed blender, combine the pitted and peeled avocado, unsweetened almond milk, honey, unsweetened cocoa powder, vanilla extract, and a pinch of salt.
2. Blend the ingredients until the mixture is smooth and creamy, scraping down the sides as needed.
3. Transfer the avocado pudding to individual serving bowls or ramekins.
4. Chill the avocado pudding in the refrigerator for at least 30 minutes before serving.

Pistachio Cranberry Dark Chocolate Bark

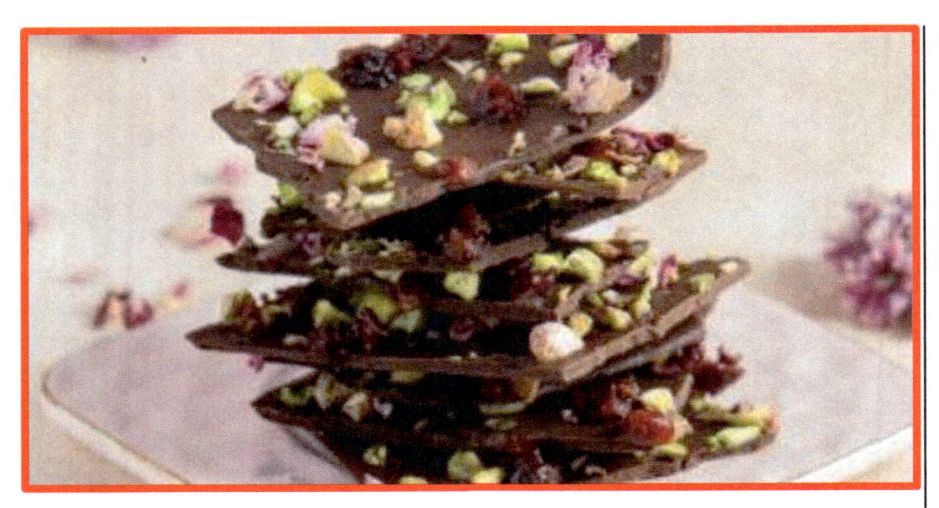

Time of Prep: 15 minutes
Cook Time: 20 minutes
Serving Size: 12 servings

Nutritional Information (per serving):
- Calories: 90
- Protein: 1g
- Fat: 6g
- Carbohydrates: 8g

Ingredients:

- 4 oz dark chocolate (70% cocoa or higher), chopped
- 1/4 cup shelled pistachios, chopped
- 1/4 cup dried cranberries
- 1 tsp coconut oil (optional)

Instructions:

1. Line a baking sheet with parchment paper.
2. In a microwave-safe bowl, combine the chopped dark chocolate and coconut oil (if using). Microwave in 30-second intervals, stirring between each interval, until the chocolate is melted and smooth.
3. Pour the melted chocolate onto the prepared baking sheet, spreading it into an even layer.
4. Sprinkle the chopped pistachios and dried cranberries evenly over the top of the chocolate.
5. Refrigerate the chocolate bark for 15-20 minutes, or until it has hardened completely.

6. Break the chocolate bark into irregular pieces and serve.

Cast Iron Mango and Peach Cobbler

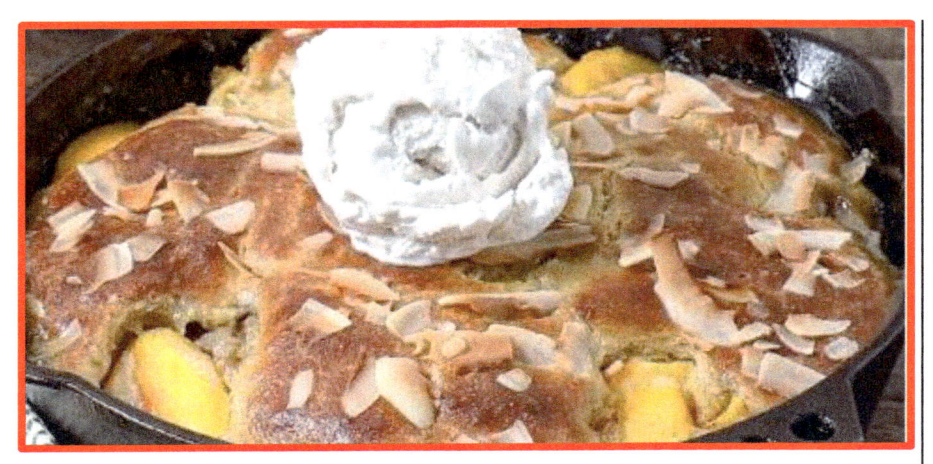

Time of Prep: 20 minutes
Cook Time: 30 minutes
Serving Size: 6 servings

Nutritional Information (per serving):
- Calories: 250
- Protein: 3g
- Fat: 8g
- Carbohydrates: 40g

Ingredients:

- 2 cups sliced fresh or frozen mango
- 2 cups sliced fresh or frozen peaches
- 1/4 cup honey
- 1 tsp ground cinnamon
- 1 cup whole wheat flour
- 1/2 cup rolled oats
- 2 tbsp brown sugar
- 1 tsp baking powder
- 1/4 tsp salt
- 4 tbsp unsalted butter, cubed

Instructions:

1. Preheat your oven to 375°F (190°C).
2. In a 9-inch cast iron skillet, combine the sliced mango, sliced peaches, honey, and ground cinnamon. Stir to mix well.

3. In a medium bowl, whisk together the whole wheat flour, rolled oats, brown sugar, baking powder, and salt.
4. Cut the unsalted butter into the dry ingredients using a fork or pastry cutter until the mixture resembles coarse crumbs.
5. Sprinkle the oat topping evenly over the fruit mixture in the cast iron skillet.
6. Bake the cobbler in the preheated oven for 25-30 minutes, or until the topping is golden brown and the fruit is bubbly.
7. Allow the cobbler to cool for 10-15 minutes before serving.

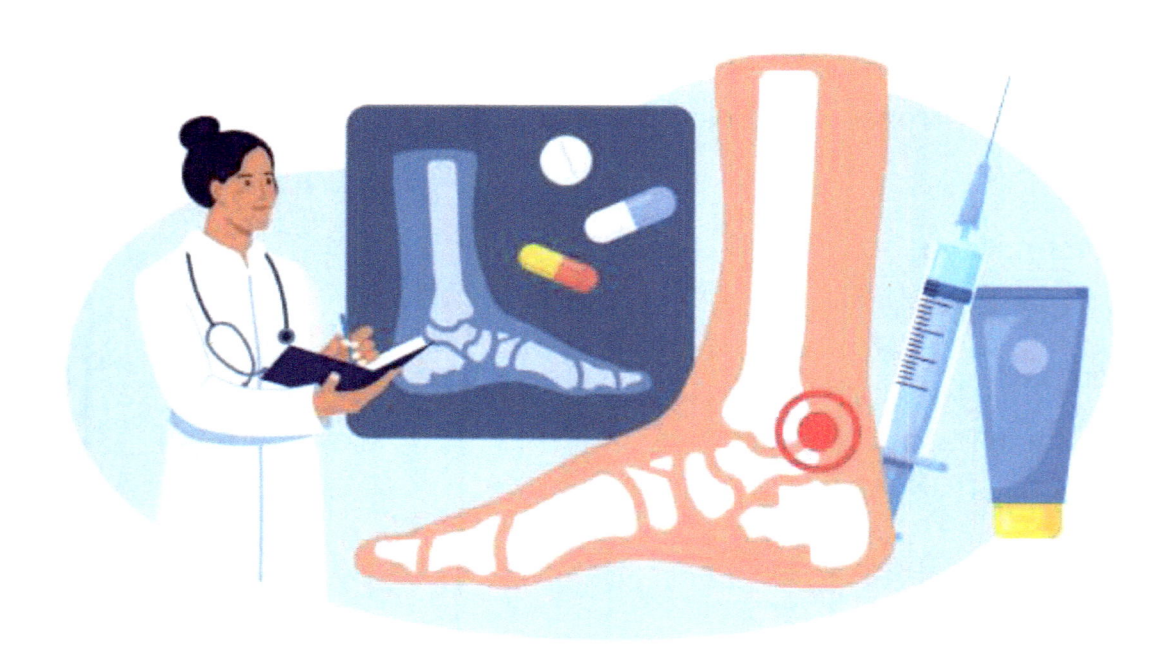

Chapter 9: Maintaining a Healthy Weight for Gout Control

The Prevalence of Gout in Older Adults

Gout is a common form of inflammatory arthritis that disproportionately affects the elderly population. As people age, the risk of developing gout increases due to factors such as decreased kidney function, changes in hormone levels, and the accumulation of comorbidities. Approximately 4% of adults over the age of 65 in the United States are affected by gout, making it a significant health concern for seniors.

There are several factors that contribute to the higher prevalence of gout in older adults:

- Changes in metabolism: As we age, our bodies become less efficient at processing purines, which can lead to higher uric acid levels.
- Underlying health conditions: Conditions like high blood pressure, obesity, and diabetes are more common in older adults and can also contribute to gout development.
- Medications: Certain medications, such as diuretics used for blood pressure control, can increase uric acid levels.

If you're an older adult experiencing sudden joint pain, it's important to see a doctor to get a proper diagnosis and discuss treatment options. Early diagnosis and management can help prevent future gout attacks and improve overall well-being.

Maintaining Healthy Weight

Maintaining a healthy weight is crucial for seniors managing gout. Excess weight, particularly around the midsection, can increase the risk of gout flare-ups and exacerbate joint pain and inflammation. Excess body weight can lead to higher levels of uric acid in the blood, which is the primary driver of gout. By achieving and maintaining a healthy weight, seniors can effectively reduce the burden of gout and improve their overall quality of life.

The key importance of weight management for gout control are:

1. Excess weight, particularly around the midsection, can increase the risk of gout flare-ups and exacerbate joint pain and inflammation.

2. The prevalence of gout is higher in individuals with obesity compared to those with normal weight. By age 65, 13.3% of men and 6.2% of women with obesity had a history of gout, compared to 9.0% of men and 3.3% of women with normal weight.

3. Studies have found that weight gain is strongly associated with an increased risk of developing gout. Gaining weight over adulthood was associated with a higher risk of incident gout.

4. Conversely, weight loss has been shown to be beneficial for gout management. A review of studies found that losing 7.7 pounds (3.5 kg) or more may reduce gout attacks. Those whose BMI decreased by 5% had 39% lower odds of gout flare-ups.

5. Hypothetical scenarios suggest that preventing weight gain or maintaining a normal weight from early adulthood to midlife could avert a significant proportion of gout cases in the population.

The search results clearly highlight that maintaining a healthy weight and avoiding weight gain are crucial for effectively managing gout and reducing the risk of gout flare-ups in older adults. Weight loss, particularly fat loss, can provide significant benefits for individuals with gout and concomitant obesity.

Safe and Effective Weight Loss Strategies for Seniors

When it comes to weight loss for seniors with gout, it's essential to adopt a balanced and sustainable approach. Crash diets or extreme calorie restriction can be harmful and may lead to nutrient deficiencies. Instead, focus on making gradual, long-term lifestyle changes that incorporate a nutrient-dense, gout-friendly diet and regular physical activity.

Some effective weight loss strategies for seniors with gout include:

1. Adopting a Gout-Friendly Diet:

- Focus on consuming low-purine foods, such as fruits, vegetables, whole grains, and lean proteins.
- Limit or avoid high-purine foods, such as red meat, seafood, and sugary beverages.
- Incorporate plenty of water and other hydrating fluids to support kidney function and uric acid excretion.

2. Engaging in Regular Physical Activity:

- Participate in low-impact exercises, such as swimming, cycling, or gentle strength training, to improve joint function and support weight management without exacerbating gout-related pain.
- Work with a healthcare provider or physical therapist to develop a personalized exercise plan that accommodates any joint limitations or mobility challenges.

3. Seeking Professional Guidance:

- Consult with a registered dietitian or healthcare provider to create a safe and effective weight loss plan that considers your individual health needs and gout management goals.
- Regularly monitor your progress and adjust your plan as needed to ensure sustainable weight loss and gout control.

By adopting a comprehensive approach to weight management, seniors with gout can take an active role in managing their condition, reducing the risk of flare-ups, and improving their overall health and well-being.

Safe and effective weight loss strategies for seniors

Losing weight safely and effectively is important for everyone, but especially for seniors with gout. Here's a breakdown of some key strategies, considering any potential differences between senior men and women:

1. Portion Control:

General Tip: Focus on mindful eating and pay attention to your body's hunger cues. Stop eating when you feel comfortably full, not stuffed.

Senior Women: Smaller portion sizes might be appropriate due to potentially lower calorie needs compared to men. Using smaller plates can be a helpful visual cue.

Senior Men: While portion control is still important, men may require slightly larger portions due to typically higher calorie needs.

2. Choose Low-Calorie, Nutrient-Dense Foods:

General Tip: Fill your plate with fruits, vegetables, and whole grains. These foods are packed with vitamins, minerals, and fiber, keeping you feeling fuller for longer with fewer calories.

Both Seniors: Opt for lean protein sources like grilled chicken, fish, or beans to feel satisfied without excess fat.

3. Integrate More Fruits and Vegetables into Meals:

General Tip: Aim for a rainbow on your plate! Include a variety of colorful fruits and vegetables at each meal and snack. They're naturally low in calories and high in water content, aiding in weight loss and overall health.

Both Seniors: Experiment with different recipes and cooking methods to keep things interesting. Roasting, steaming, or grilling vegetables are healthy preparation options.

4. Limit Sugary Drinks and Processed Foods:

General Tip: Sugary drinks like soda and processed foods are packed with empty calories and offer little nutritional value. They can contribute to weight gain and worsen inflammation, a potential gout trigger.

Both Seniors: Opt for water or unsweetened tea/coffee instead of sugary drinks. Read food labels carefully and choose options lower in added sugar and processed ingredients.

Additional Considerations for Seniors:

Strength Training: While exercise is crucial, strength training can be especially beneficial for senior men to maintain muscle mass, which can help with metabolism. However, both men and women can benefit from gentle strength exercises tailored to their abilities.

Bone Health: Senior women are more susceptible to osteoporosis. Include calcium-rich foods like yogurt and low-fat dairy products (if tolerated) in their diet to support bone health alongside weight loss efforts.

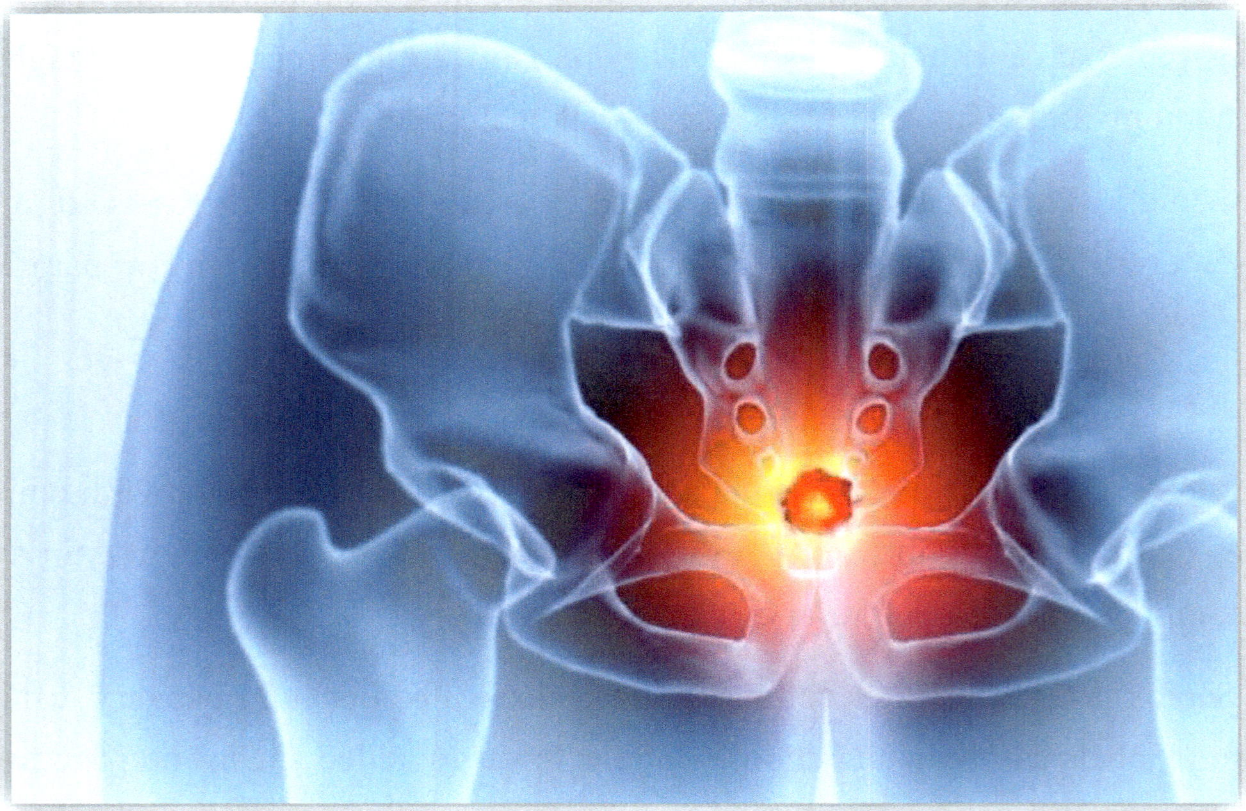

Chapter 10: Exercise and Physicala Activity

While it might seem counterintuitive to move when your joints hurt, the right kinds of activities can actually reduce pain, improve mobility, and help prevent future gout attacks.

Why Exercise Matters

- **Weight Management:** Exercise helps you maintain a healthy weight, which is crucial for gout management. Excess weight puts extra stress on your joints and increases uric acid production.

- **Reduced Inflammation:** Regular physical activity can help lower inflammation throughout your body, including in your joints.

- **Improved Circulation:** Exercise improves blood flow, which helps to remove uric acid crystals from your joints.

- **Stronger Joints and Muscles:** Strengthening the muscles around your joints provides better support and stability, reducing strain and pain.

- **Enhanced Mood:** Exercise releases endorphins, which have mood-boosting effects and can help you cope with the challenges of gout.

Gout-Friendly Exercise Options

- **Low-Impact Activities:** These are gentle on your joints and are a great starting point.
    - **Walking:** Start with short walks and gradually increase the duration and intensity.
    - **Water Aerobics:** The buoyancy of water supports your joints while providing resistance for a great workout.
    - **Swimming:** Swimming is an excellent full-body exercise that's easy on the joints.

- **Cycling:** Whether outdoors or on a stationary bike, cycling is a low-impact way to improve cardiovascular health.
- **Yoga:** Gentle yoga poses can improve flexibility, balance, and strength.
- **Tai Chi:** This slow, flowing practice can enhance range of motion and reduce stress.

Staying Active with Joint Limitations

- **Listen to Your Body:** Pay attention to your body's signals and don't push yourself too hard, especially during a gout flare.
- **Start Slowly:** Begin with shorter sessions and gradually increase the duration and intensity of your workouts.
- **Modify Exercises:** If an exercise causes pain, modify it or find an alternative.
- **Stay Consistent:** Aim for at least 30 minutes of moderate-intensity exercise most days of the week.
- **Warm Up and Cool Down:** Always warm up before exercise and cool down afterward to prevent injury.
- **Consult Your Doctor:** Talk to your doctor or a physical therapist to develop an exercise plan that's safe and effective for you.

Key Takeaway

Exercise is a valuable tool for managing gout and improving your overall quality of life. By choosing activities that are gentle on your joints and listening to your body, you can stay active, reduce pain, and enjoy the many benefits of movement.

Chapter 11: Hydration and Lifestyle Habits for Healthy Aging with Gout

This chapter explores the crucial role that hydration and other lifestyle factors play in managing gout and promoting overall well-being, especially for seniors. By understanding the impact of these habits, you can take proactive steps to reduce gout flares, improve your quality of life, and support healthy aging.

Importance of Staying Hydrated for Gout Sufferers

Water is essential for life, and it's especially crucial for people with gout. Staying properly hydrated helps your kidneys flush out excess uric acid, which is the main culprit behind gout attacks.

- **How Dehydration Contributes to Gout:** When you're dehydrated, your body conserves water, and this can lead to a buildup of uric acid in your bloodstream. This increases the risk of uric acid crystals forming in your joints, triggering painful inflammation and gout flares.
- **Daily Fluid Intake:** Aim to drink plenty of water throughout the day. A good general guideline is to drink at least 8 glasses of water per day, but individual needs may vary depending on factors like activity level, climate, and overall health.
- **Hydrating Beverages:** Water is the best choice for hydration, but you can also include other beverages like herbal tea, diluted fruit juice, and low-fat milk.
- **Monitoring Hydration:** Pay attention to the color of your urine. Pale yellow urine is a good indicator of adequate hydration, while dark yellow urine suggests you need to drink more fluids.

The Impact of Alcohol and Sugary Drinks on Gout

Certain beverages can worsen gout symptoms and should be limited or avoided:

- **Alcohol:** Alcohol, particularly beer, is high in purines and can interfere with your body's ability to eliminate uric acid. It can also trigger dehydration. If you choose to drink alcohol, do so in moderation and opt for lower-purine options like wine.
- **Sugary Drinks:** Sugary drinks like soda and some fruit juices are often high in fructose, which can increase uric acid production and contribute to gout flares. Choose water, unsweetened tea, or diluted fruit juice instead.

Stress Management Techniques for Seniors with Gout

Stress can play a role in triggering gout flares. Finding healthy ways to manage stress is important for both physical and mental well-being.

- **Relaxation Techniques:** Practice relaxation techniques like deep breathing, meditation, or yoga to help calm your mind and body.
- **Physical Activity:** Engage in regular physical activity that you enjoy, as exercise can help reduce stress and improve mood.
- **Hobbies and Social Connections:** Spend time pursuing hobbies and interests, and maintain strong social connections to foster a sense of purpose and belonging.
- **Seek Support:** If you're struggling with stress, don't hesitate to seek support from a therapist, counselor, or support group.

Importance of Good Sleep for Overall Health

Quality sleep is essential for overall health and can also impact gout management.

- **Sleep and Inflammation:** Lack of sleep can contribute to increased inflammation throughout the body, which can worsen gout symptoms.

- **Sleep Hygiene:** Practice good sleep hygiene habits, such as maintaining a regular sleep schedule, creating a relaxing bedtime routine, and ensuring a comfortable sleep environment.

- **Addressing Sleep Issues:** If you have chronic sleep problems, consult your doctor to rule out any underlying medical conditions.

By adopting healthy lifestyle habits, including staying hydrated, limiting alcohol and sugary drinks, managing stress, and prioritizing good sleep, you can significantly improve your gout management and support your overall health and well-being as you age.

28-Day Meal Plan

Day	Breakfast	Lunch	Dinner	Snack
1	Greek Yogurt with Fresh Fruit, Chia Seeds & Almonds (350 kcal)	Whole Grain Chicken Spinach Mushroom Flatbread (450 kcal)	Marinated Baked Salmon with Herb-Roasted Vegetables (500 kcal)	Fruit Salad with Honey-Lime Dressing (150 kcal)
2	Avocado Toast with Tomato, Basil, and Smoked Salmon (400 kcal)	Salad with Cheese, Avocado, and Hard-Boiled Egg (400 kcal)	Lean Chicken and Broccoli Stir-Fry (450 kcal)	Greek Yogurt Dip with Crunchy Veggies (200 kcal)
3	Grapefruit and Cottage Cheese with Mixed Nuts (300 kcal)	Turkey, Avocado, and Tomato Wrap with Spinach (400 kcal)	Flavorful Lentil and Sweet Potato Curry (450 kcal)	Caprese Skewers with Balsamic Drizzle (150 kcal)
4	Whole Wheat Toast with Natural Peanut Butter, Banana, and Chia Seeds (350 kcal)	Vegetable Omelet with Feta Cheese (350 kcal)	Lean Beef and Barley Soup (400 kcal)	Quinoa and Feta Stuffed Bell Peppers (250 kcal)
5	Spinach and Feta Stuffed Mushrooms with Quinoa (400 kcal)	Whole Wheat Mac 'n Cheese with Ham and Broccoli (500 kcal)	Stuffed Bell Peppers with Turkey and Quinoa (500 kcal)	Cucumber Avocado Rolls with Herbs (100 kcal)
6	Baked Oatmeal with Blueberries, Almonds, and Greek Yogurt (400 kcal)	Roast Chicken with Garlic Potatoes and Glazed Carrots (550 kcal)	Tuna Salad Lettuce Wraps with Crunchy Vegetables (350 kcal)	Crispy Baked Sweet Potato Fries (200 kcal)
7	Veggie Omelet with Goat Cheese and Fresh Herbs (350 kcal)	Baked Salmon with Quinoa and Steamed Broccoli (500 kcal)	Baked Cod with Almond-Herb Topping (450 kcal)	Edamame with Lemon Pepper Seasoning (150 kcal)
8	Greek Yogurt with Fresh Fruit, Chia	Beef & Barley Soup with Leafy	Vegetable Frittata with Feta and	Fruit Salad with Honey-Lime

	Seeds & Almonds (350 kcal)	Greens (400 kcal)	Spinach (450 kcal)	Dressing (150 kcal)
9	Avocado Toast with Tomato, Basil, and Smoked Salmon (400 kcal)	Whole Grain Ham and Cheese Panini (450 kcal)	Turkey Meatballs with Whole Wheat Pasta and Steamed Broccoli (500 kcal)	Greek Yogurt Dip with Crunchy Veggies (200 kcal)
10	Grapefruit and Cottage Cheese with Mixed Nuts (300 kcal)	Salad with Cheese, Avocado, and Hard-Boiled Egg (400 kcal)	Creamy Butternut Squash Soup with Toasted Pumpkin Seeds (400 kcal)	Spiced Roasted Chickpeas (150 kcal)
11	Whole Wheat Toast with Natural Peanut Butter, Banana, and Chia Seeds (350 kcal)	Turkey, Avocado, and Tomato Wrap with Spinach (400 kcal)	Lean Beef and Barley Soup (400 kcal)	Mango Salsa with Whole Grain Pita Chips (200 kcal)
12	Egg White Veggie Frittata with Kale and Fresh Herbs (350 kcal)	Whole Wheat Mac 'n Cheese with Ham and Broccoli (500 kcal)	Marinated Baked Salmon with Herb-Roasted Vegetables (500 kcal)	Cucumber Avocado Rolls with Herbs (100 kcal)
13	Baked Oatmeal with Blueberries, Almonds, and Greek Yogurt (400 kcal)	Hearty Beef and Root Vegetable Stew (500 kcal)	Lean Chicken and Broccoli Stir-Fry (450 kcal)	Crispy Baked Sweet Potato Fries (200 kcal)
14	Overnight Oats with Berries, Walnuts, and Protein Powder (400 kcal)	Baked Salmon with Quinoa and Steamed Broccoli (500 kcal)	Flavorful Lentil and Sweet Potato Curry (450 kcal)	Edamame with Lemon Pepper Seasoning (150 kcal)
15	Quinoa Porridge with Cinnamon, Apples, and Flaxseed (350 kcal)	Whole Grain Chicken Spinach Mushroom Flatbread (450 kcal)	Stuffed Bell Peppers with Turkey and Quinoa (500 kcal)	Fruit Salad with Honey-Lime Dressing (150 kcal)
16	Greek Yogurt with Fresh Fruit, Chia Seeds & Almonds (350 kcal)	Beef & Barley Soup with Leafy Greens (400 kcal)	Tuna Salad Lettuce Wraps with Crunchy Vegetables (350 kcal)	Greek Yogurt Dip with Crunchy Veggies (200 kcal)

17	Avocado Toast with Tomato, Basil, and Smoked Salmon (400 kcal)	Salad with Cheese, Avocado, and Hard-Boiled Egg (400 kcal)	Baked Cod with Almond-Herb Topping (450 kcal)	Caprese Skewers with Balsamic Drizzle (150 kcal)
18	Grapefruit and Cottage Cheese with Mixed Nuts (300 kcal)	Turkey, Avocado, and Tomato Wrap with Spinach (400 kcal)	Vegetable Frittata with Feta and Spinach (450 kcal)	Quinoa and Feta Stuffed Bell Peppers (250 kcal)
19	Whole Wheat Toast with Natural Peanut Butter, Banana, and Chia Seeds (350 kcal)	Vegetable Omelet with Feta Cheese (350 kcal)	Turkey Meatballs with Whole Wheat Pasta and Steamed Broccoli (500 kcal)	Cucumber Avocado Rolls with Herbs (100 kcal)
20	Spinach and Feta Stuffed Mushrooms with Quinoa (400 kcal)	Whole Wheat Mac 'n Cheese with Ham and Broccoli (500 kcal)	Creamy Butternut Squash Soup with Toasted Pumpkin Seeds (400 kcal)	Spiced Roasted Chickpeas (150 kcal)
21	Egg White Veggie Frittata with Kale and Fresh Herbs (350 kcal)	Roast Chicken with Garlic Potatoes and Glazed Carrots (550 kcal)	Lean Beef and Barley Soup (400 kcal)	Mango Salsa with Whole Grain Pita Chips (200 kcal)
22	Baked Oatmeal with Blueberries, Almonds, and Greek Yogurt (400 kcal)	Baked Salmon with Quinoa and Steamed Broccoli (500 kcal)	Marinated Baked Salmon with Herb-Roasted Vegetables (500 kcal)	Easy Applesauce (Dessert) (100 kcal)
23	Overnight Oats with Berries, Walnuts, and Protein Powder (400 kcal)	Hearty Beef and Root Vegetable Stew (500 kcal)	Lean Chicken and Broccoli Stir-Fry (450 kcal)	Edamame with Lemon Pepper Seasoning (150 kcal)
24	Quinoa Porridge with Cinnamon, Apples, and Flaxseed (350 kcal)	Whole Grain Chicken Spinach Mushroom Flatbread (450 kcal)	Flavorful Lentil and Sweet Potato Curry (450 kcal)	Berry Cherry Smoothie (Dessert) (150 kcal)
25	Greek Yogurt with Fresh Fruit, Chia	Beef & Barley Soup with Leafy	Stuffed Bell Peppers with	Fruit Salad with Honey-Lime

	Seeds & Almonds (350 kcal)	Greens (400 kcal)	Turkey and Quinoa (500 kcal)	Dressing (150 kcal)
26	Avocado Toast with Tomato, Basil, and Smoked Salmon (400 kcal)	Salad with Cheese, Avocado, and Hard-Boiled Egg (400 kcal)	Tuna Salad Lettuce Wraps with Crunchy Vegetables (350 kcal)	Greek Yogurt Dip with Crunchy Veggies (200 kcal)
27	Grapefruit and Cottage Cheese with Mixed Nuts (300 kcal)	Turkey, Avocado, and Tomato Wrap with Spinach (400 kcal)	Baked Cod with Almond-Herb Topping (450 kcal)	Chocolate Covered Strawberries (Dessert) (150 kcal)
28	Whole Wheat Toast with Natural Peanut Butter, Banana, and Chia Seeds (350 kcal)	Vegetable Omelet with Feta Cheese (350 kcal)	Vegetable Frittata with Feta and Spinach (450 kcal)	Quinoa and Feta Stuffed Bell Peppers (250 kcal)

Gout-Friendly Weekly Shopping List

Week 1

- **Produce:**
  - Bananas
  - Berries
  - Avocado
  - Tomato
  - Basil
  - Smoked salmon
  - Grapefruit
  - Cottage cheese
  - Mixed nuts
  - Whole wheat bread
  - Natural peanut butter
  - Spinach
  - Feta cheese
  - Quinoa
  - Blueberries
  - Almonds
  - Goat cheese
  - Overnight oats
  - Walnuts
  - Protein powder
  - Cinnamon
  - Apples
  - Flaxseed
  - Egg whites
  - Kale
  - Fresh herbs
- **Protein:**
  - Chicken breast
  - Ground beef
  - Lentil
  - Sweet potato
  - Turkey
  - Tuna
  - Cod
  - Turkey meatballs
  - Tofu (optional)
- **Dairy:**
  - Greek yogurt
  - Cheese
  - Milk (if needed)
- **Grains:**
  - Whole wheat flour
  - Whole wheat pasta
  - Brown rice
  - Quinoa
  - Oats
- **Pantry staples:**
  - Olive oil
  - Vegetable oil
  - Butter
  - Salt
  - Pepper
  - Garlic powder
  - Onion powder
  - Paprika
  - Cumin
  - Coriander
  - Curry powder
  - Soy sauce

- Balsamic vinegar
- Honey
- Lemon juice
- Worcestershire sauce
- Mayonnaise
- Mustard
- Ketchup
- BBQ sauce
- Hot sauce
- Chili powder
- Oregano
- Thyme
- Rosemary
- Parsley
- Cilantro
- Ginger
- Garlic
- Onion

Week 2
- **Produce:**
  - Oranges
  - Pears
  - Broccoli
  - Carrots
  - Celery
  - Red onion
  - Bell peppers
  - Cucumbers
  - Mushrooms
  - Romaine lettuce
  - Spinach
  - Tomatoes
  - Black beans
  - Corn
  - Green peas
- **Protein:**
  - Chicken breast
  - Ground beef
  - Salmon
  - Shrimp
  - Tofu (optional)
  - Lentils
  - Black beans
  - Chickpeas
  - Eggs
- **Dairy:**
  - Greek yogurt
  - Cheese
  - Milk (if needed)
- **Grains:**
  - Whole wheat flour
  - Whole wheat pasta
  - Brown rice
  - Quinoa
  - Oats
- **Pantry staples:**
  - Olive oil
  - Vegetable oil
  - Butter
  - Salt
  - Pepper
  - Garlic powder
  - Onion powder
  - Paprika
  - Cumin
  - Coriander
  - Curry powder
  - Soy sauce
  - Balsamic vinegar
  - Honey
  - Lemon juice
  - Worcestershire sauce
  - Mayonnaise
  - Mustard
  - Ketchup
  - BBQ sauce
  - Hot sauce
  - Chili powder
  - Oregano
  - Thyme
  - Rosemary
  - Parsley
  - Cilantro
  - Ginger
  - Garlic
  - Onion

Week 3
- **Produce:**
  - Apples
  - Pears
  - Grapes
  - Strawberries
  - Bananas
  - Sweet potatoes
  - Butternut squash
  - Carrots
  - Celery
  - Red onion
  - Bell peppers
  - Cucumbers
  - Mushrooms
  - Romaine lettuce
  - Spinach
  - Tomatoes
- **Protein:**
  - Chicken breast
  - Ground beef
  - Salmon
  - Shrimp
  - Tofu (optional)
  - Lentils
  - Black beans
  - Chickpeas
  - Eggs
- **Dairy:**
  - Greek yogurt
  - Cheese
  - Milk (if needed)
- **Grains:**
  - Whole wheat flour

- Whole wheat pasta
- Brown rice
- Quinoa
- Oats
- **Pantry staples:**
  - Olive oil
  - Vegetable oil
  - Butter
  - Salt
  - Pepper
  - Garlic powder
  - Onion powder
  - Paprika
  - Cumin
  - Coriander
  - Curry powder
  - Soy sauce
  - Balsamic vinegar
  - Honey
  - Lemon juice
  - Worcestershire sauce
  - Mayonnaise
  - Mustard
  - Ketchup
  - BBQ sauce
  - Hot sauce
  - Chili powder
  - Oregano
  - Thyme
  - Rosemary
  - Parsley
  - Cilantro
  - Ginger
  - Garlic
  - Onion

Week 4

- **Produce:**
  - Oranges
  - Grapefruit
  - Mangoes
  - Strawberries
  - Bananas
  - Sweet potatoes
  - Butternut squash
  - Carrots
  - Celery
  - Red onion
  - Bell peppers
  - Cucumbers
  - Mushrooms
  - Romaine lettuce
  - Spinach
  - Tomatoes
- **Protein:**
  - Chicken breast
  - Ground beef
  - Salmon
  - Shrimp
  - Tofu (optional)
  - Lentils
  - Black beans
  - Chickpeas
  - Eggs
- **Dairy:**
  - Greek yogurt
  - Cheese
  - Milk (if needed)
- **Grains:**
  - Whole wheat flour
  - Whole wheat pasta
  - Brown rice
  - Quinoa
  - Oats
- **Pantry staples:**
  - Olive oil
  - Vegetable oil
  - Butter
  - Salt
  - Pepper
  - Garlic powder
  - Onion powder
  - Paprika
  - Cumin
  - Coriander
  - Curry powder
  - Soy sauce
  - Balsamic vinegar
  - Honey
  - Lemon juice
  - Worcestershire sauce
  - Mayonnaise
  - Mustard
  - Ketchup
  - BBQ sauce
  - Hot sauce
  - Chili powder
  - Oregano
  - Thyme
  - Rosemary
  - Parsley
  - Cilantro
  - Ginger
  - Garlic
  - Onion

Bonus Section

The Gout-Friendly Plate: Your Guide to Delicious Living

This special bonus section is your roadmap to navigating the world of food with gout. We've compiled a comprehensive list of foods, categorized by their purine content, to help you understand what to enjoy freely, what to savor in moderation, and what to limit. More than just a list, this guide empowers you to take control of your plate and your health. Discover the joy of eating well while managing gout, and unlock a life filled with flavor and vitality!

Your Green Light Foods: Enjoy These Freely!

These are your "**green light**" foods—naturally **low in purines** and packed with vitamins, minerals, and antioxidants to support your overall health and help keep gout at bay.

Why These Foods Are Great for Gout

When your body breaks down purines, it creates uric acid. High levels of uric acid can lead to painful gout flares. The foods in this list are naturally low in purines, meaning they won't contribute to a buildup of uric acid in your body.

Fill Your Plate with These!

- **Fruits:**
    - **A rainbow of options:** Enjoy a variety of colorful fruits like berries, cherries, citrus fruits, melons, and tropical fruits.
    - **Benefits:** Fruits are packed with vitamins, minerals, and antioxidants that fight inflammation and support overall health. Cherries, in particular, may help lower uric acid levels.

- **Vegetables:**
    - **Load up on veggies:** Include plenty of leafy greens, cruciferous vegetables, root vegetables, and other colorful choices in your meals.
    - **Benefits:** Vegetables are low in calories and high in fiber, which can help you maintain a healthy weight and promote good digestion.

- **Grains:**
  - **Choose whole grains:** Opt for whole grains like brown rice, quinoa, oats, and whole wheat bread and pasta.
  - **Benefits:** Whole grains provide sustained energy, fiber, and important nutrients.
- **Dairy:**
  - **Low-fat is best:** Enjoy low-fat or non-fat milk, yogurt, and cheese.
  - **Benefits:** Dairy products provide calcium and vitamin D for strong bones.
- **Protein:**
  - **Plant-based power:** Include plenty of plant-based proteins like tofu, tempeh, lentils, beans, and peas.
  - **Eggs in moderation:** Enjoy eggs in moderation (around 4-6 per week).
  - **Fish choices:** Opt for low-purine fish like salmon, cod, and tuna (in moderation).
  - **Benefits:** Protein is essential for building and repairing tissues. Plant-based proteins are particularly beneficial for gout, as they are naturally low in purines.
- **Healthy Fats:**
  - **Good fats are essential:** Include healthy fats in moderation, such as olive oil, avocados, and nuts and seeds.
  - **Benefits:** Healthy fats support heart health, brain function, and overall well-being.

Important Reminders

- **Variety is key:** Eat a variety of foods from this list to ensure you're getting a wide range of nutrients.
- **Hydration matters:** Drink plenty of water throughout the day to help flush out uric acid.
- **Listen to your body:** Pay attention to how your body responds to different foods and adjust your intake accordingly.

This "green light" list is your foundation for a delicious and gout-friendly diet. Enjoy these foods freely and build a foundation for a healthier, happier you!

Moderate-Purine Foods: Finding the Balance

This section is all about understanding those "in-between" foods—the ones that offer valuable nutrition but also contain a moderate amount of purines. Here's the key: It's not about avoiding these foods entirely, but rather enjoying them mindfully as part of a balanced approach to managing gout.

Why Moderation Matters

Purines are natural compounds found in many foods. When your body breaks down purines, it produces uric acid. For some people, especially those with gout, the body can struggle to eliminate excess uric acid. This can lead to a buildup of uric acid crystals in the joints, causing painful inflammation and gout flares.

Moderate-purine foods won't necessarily trigger a gout attack if you enjoy them in reasonable portions and frequencies. However, overdoing it might increase your risk. That's why portion control and variety are essential.

Foods to Enjoy in Moderation

- **Protein:**
  - **Lean meats:** Chicken, turkey, duck (limit to 4-6 ounces per day)
    - **Tip:** Choose lean cuts of meat and trim away visible fat. Removing poultry skin can also help reduce purine content.
  - **Fish:** Tuna, halibut, snapper (limit to 4-6 ounces per day)
    - **Tip:** Opt for fresh or frozen fish whenever possible, as canned varieties may be higher in purines.
- **Vegetables:**
  - **Asparagus** (limit to ½ cup per day)
  - **Cauliflower** (limit to ½ cup per day)
  - **Spinach** (limit to ½ cup per day) - *While spinach is a nutritional powerhouse, it's best enjoyed in moderation due to its oxalate*

content, which can contribute to kidney stones in some individuals.

- **Mushrooms** (limit to ½ cup per day)
- **Green peas** (limit to ½ cup per day)
- **Beans, peas, and lentils** (limit to 1 cup per day) - *These legumes are excellent sources of protein and fiber, but it's best to limit their intake to 1 cup per day.*

Tips for Managing Moderate-Purine Foods

- **Variety is Your Friend:** Don't eat the same moderate-purine food every day. Mix it up to ensure a balanced intake of nutrients and minimize the risk of excess purines.
- **Cooking Methods Matter:** Grilling or broiling meats can create purine-rich compounds. Consider baking, roasting, or stewing as healthier alternatives.
- **Hydration is Essential:** Drink plenty of water throughout the day, especially when consuming moderate-purine foods. Water helps flush out uric acid and can reduce your risk of gout flares.
- **Listen to Your Body:** Pay attention to how your body responds to different foods in this category. If you notice any discomfort or increased gout symptoms after eating a particular food, consider reducing your intake or avoiding it altogether.

The Bottom Line

Moderate-purine foods can be part of a healthy and enjoyable diet for people with gout. The key is moderation, variety, and mindful eating. By following these guidelines, you can savor the flavors and benefits of these foods while keeping your gout symptoms under control.

High-Purine Foods: Proceed with Caution

This section focuses on foods that are particularly high in purines. While not completely forbidden, these are the ones that require the most careful consideration and portion control for those managing gout.

Understanding the Risks

High-purine foods can significantly raise uric acid levels in your bloodstream. For people with gout, this can increase the likelihood of painful gout attacks. While everyone's tolerance is different, it's generally wise to limit these foods or avoid them altogether.

Foods to Limit or Avoid

- **Organ Meats:**
    - Liver
    - Kidney
    - Sweetbreads (thymus or pancreas)
    - **Why they're high in purines:** Organ meats are naturally concentrated sources of purines.
- **Red Meat:**
    - Beef
    - Lamb
    - Pork
    - Veal
    - Venison
    - **Why they're high in purines:** Red meats contain higher levels of purines compared to poultry or fish.
- **Certain Seafood:**
    - Anchovies
    - Sardines
    - Mussels
    - Scallops
    - Herring
    - Trout (some varieties)
    - **Why they're high in purines:** These types of seafood are particularly purine-rich.
- **Alcohol:**
    - Beer (especially)
    - Distilled liquors (whiskey, vodka, gin)
    - **Why alcohol is a concern:** Alcohol can interfere with your body's ability to eliminate uric acid, leading to a buildup in your system. Beer is particularly high in purines.
- **Sugary Drinks:**

- Soda
- Fruit juices (some)
- **Why they're problematic:** Sugary drinks are often high in fructose, which can break down into uric acid and contribute to gout flares.

- **High-Fructose Corn Syrup:**
  - Found in many processed foods and drinks
  - **Why it's a concern:** High-fructose corn syrup is a concentrated form of fructose, which can increase uric acid production.

Important Considerations

- **Individual Tolerance:** Some people with gout may be more sensitive to high-purine foods than others. Pay attention to your body's signals and adjust your intake accordingly.
- **Occasional Indulgences:** It's okay to enjoy a small portion of a high-purine food occasionally, but be mindful of the frequency and portion size.
- **Healthy Swaps:** Look for lower-purine alternatives to your favorite high-purine foods. For example, instead of red meat, try chicken or fish.
- **Hydration:** Always drink plenty of water, especially if you do consume high-purine foods, to help flush out uric acid.
- **Consult Your Doctor:** If you have any concerns about your diet or gout management, talk to your doctor or a registered dietitian. They can provide personalized guidance and support.

Conclusion

Living with gout doesn't mean you have to sacrifice flavor or enjoyment when it comes to food. This book has provided you with the knowledge and tools to take control of your diet, manage your gout symptoms, and live a vibrant, fulfilling life. By understanding the role of purines, embracing a variety of delicious low-purine foods, and adopting healthy lifestyle habits, you can reduce the frequency and severity of gout attacks and improve your overall well-being.

Remember that everyone's experience with gout is unique. Listen to your body, pay attention to how different foods make you feel, and don't hesitate to adjust your diet and lifestyle accordingly. This book is your guide, but you are the expert on your own body.

As you embark on this journey of delicious discovery and gout-friendly living, keep these key principles in mind:

- **Variety is key:** Explore a wide range of low-purine foods to ensure a balanced and enjoyable diet.
- **Hydration matters:** Drink plenty of water to help flush out excess uric acid.
- **Mindful eating:** Pay attention to portion sizes and savor each bite.
- **Move your body:** Engage in regular physical activity that you enjoy.
- **Manage stress:** Find healthy ways to cope with stress and promote relaxation.
- **Prioritize sleep:** Aim for quality sleep to support overall health and reduce inflammation.

This cookbook is more than just a collection of recipes; it's a roadmap to a healthier, happier you. Embrace the journey, savor the flavors, and enjoy the freedom of living a gout-friendly life!

A Note from the Author

Thank you for choosing "The Complete Gout-Friendly Cookbook for Seniors"! I sincerely hope that this book empowers you to take control of your gout, discover the joy of delicious, healthy eating, and live a more vibrant life.

It has been a labor of love to compile these recipes and resources, and my greatest wish is that they make a positive difference in your journey with gout. Whether you're enjoying a pain-free morning with a delicious breakfast or savoring a flavorful dinner with loved ones, I hope this cookbook becomes your trusted companion in the kitchen.

Your feedback is incredibly valuable to me. If you've found this cookbook helpful, I would be honored if you would leave an honest review on Amazon. Your review will help other seniors discover these gout-friendly recipes and resources, and it will mean the world to me to know that I've made a difference.

Thank you for joining me on this culinary adventure. Here's to your health, happiness, and a life filled with flavor!

Warmly,

Grace N. Rodney

Printed in Dunstable, United Kingdom